MED SCHOOL
UNCENSORED

MED SCHOOL UNCENSORED

the *INSIDER'S* GUIDE *to* SURVIVING ADMISSIONS, EXAMS, RESIDENCY, *and* SLEEPLESS NIGHTS *in the* CALL ROOM

RICHARD BEDDINGFIELD, M.D.

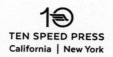

TEN SPEED PRESS
California | New York

www.crownpublishing.com
www.tenspeed.com

Ten Speed Press and the Ten Speed Press colophon are registered
trademarks of Penguin Random House LLC.

Library of Congress Cataloging-in-Publication Data

Names: Beddingfield, Richard, author.
Title: Med school uncensored : the insider's guide to surviving
admissions, exams, residency, and sleepless nights in the call room /
Richard Beddingfield, M.D.
Description: First edition. | New York : Ten Speed Press, [2017] |
Includes bibliographical references and index.
Identifiers: LCCN 2017009792 (print) | LCCN 2017014382 (ebook) |
ISBN 9780399579714 (E-book) | ISBN 9780399579707 (paperback)
Subjects: LCSH: Medical students—Vocational guidance. |
Medical students—Psychology. | Residents (Medicine)—Life skills guides.
| Medical education—Miscellanea. | BISAC: EDUCATION / Higher. |
MEDICAL / Education & Training. | MEDICAL / Test Preparation & Review.
Classification: LCC R737 (ebook) | LCC R737 .B43 2017 (print) |
DDC 610.71/55—dc23
LC record available at https://lccn.loc.gov/2017009792

Trade Paperback ISBN: 978-0-399-57970-7
eBook ISBN: 978-0-399-57971-4

Printed in the United States of America

Design by Lizzie Allen
Cover image copyright © OZMedia/Shutterstock.com

10 9 8 7 6 5 4 3 2 1

First Edition

To Laura, my lovely wife and devoted mother of Lydia and Audrey. After enduring my nine years of medical training, she was gracious enough to support my dream of writing and publishing this book.

CONTENTS

ACKNOWLEDGMENTS

I am thankful beyond words to the many people who encouraged, inspired, and educated me throughout my journey of becoming a physician, anesthesiologist, and author:

My parents, Harris and Peggy, worked tirelessly to prepare me for professional and personal success. Full recognition of their sacrifices emerged only in recent years, as I am now the proud and exhausted father of two wonderful children.

Dr. Gerald Abrams ignited within me one of the earliest flickers of interest in becoming a physician. The passion exhibited during his lectures at the University of Michigan Mini-Med School was contagious. Later, he affirmed my decision to become a physician—and encouraged me to always continue writing.

My uncle, Dr. George Beddingfield, retired thoracic surgeon and author of several novels, was immensely helpful during my initial inquiries about becoming a physician. He also never wavered in his encouragement and assistance of my literary career.

My editor, Lisa Westmoreland, designer Lizzie Allen, copyeditor Kristi Hein, and everyone else at Ten Speed Press who helped make this book a reality—and even better than I first imagined.

I cannot forget the many attending physicians, fellows, residents, and senior students who taught me the science and art of medicine. Also, the nurses, technicians, and other health care providers who taught me how to get things done.

Most of all, I am grateful to the countless patients I have encountered throughout my education and career. Each day, I continue to learn from the most rebellious ones who forgot to read the textbooks.

INTRODUCTION

Interview with a Pre-Med

It was a typical January evening in Minnesota. The air was biting cold, with temperatures well below freezing. The sun had set hours before I was done with work on my ICU rotation. I left the warmth of the hospital to meet a pre-med student at a nearby coffee shop to talk about my experiences in medical school. I've long since forgotten his name, but I remember he was a young undergrad at the University of Minnesota, studying biology. He was bright-eyed and a bit nervous about meeting a real live medical student, that being me.

On a whim, I had responded a few weeks prior to an email from a pre-med interest group asking for senior medical students to meet with randomly assigned undergrads to impart to them our vast array of experiences and wisdom gained in the four torturous years of becoming a doctor. As I knocked the snow off my boots, I thought I'd rather be home cracking open a beer than bracing myself for an hour of questions from an overly eager pre-med.

He immediately recognized me by the Minnesota sweatshirt I'd told him I would be wearing. It felt a bit like a blind date, though not one I would have been excited about. He was armed with a small notepad and pen. I paid for his coffee, but in retrospect I'm not sure why. Being a senior medical student, I had by that time accumulated massive amounts of student debt, so I'm sure he was better off financially than I was.

We picked a table in the corner, and he immediately recited a well-rehearsed introduction. He asked how far along I was in my studies, whether I had chosen my specialty, and if I knew yet where I would be going for residency.

I answered his questions and kind of got into the whole thing. I felt like a B-list celebrity, interviewed by this eager young student listening intently to my every word, recording it in his black notepad. I hammed it up a bit, waxing poetic about my circuitous decision to become a doctor, how I'd selected my medical school, what led me to my chosen specialty.

After a glowing self-introduction, I opened the floor to my interviewer. "So, what do you want to know about medical school? I'm just a few months from graduation, so I can tell you all about it, from the first week of gross anatomy to the final rotations and residency match."

I was ready to share my treasure trove of knowledge and experience. I tried to imagine his most pressing questions. He might ask about the workload in medical school, the material covered in our preclinical years, the diverse and eye-opening experiences of rotating as a student in the wards or operating rooms.

He began: "So here's what I really want to know about medical school: What MCAT score guarantees that I'll get in?"

Are you freakin' kidding me? I couldn't believe it. I was in my final year of med school, just months from graduation. I had been through it all! I had dissected a full cadaver, taken countless exams on everything from pathology to physiology, memorized every muscle and bone in the body, admitted homicidal patients in the county psychiatric ward, scrubbed in for twelve-hour heart surgeries. I had countless interesting experiences and myriad advice to impart, and *this* was his question?

I gave him some BS answer, and he continued: "What topic did you choose for your admissions essay? Are there any topics that will help someone get in?"

And the next question: "Right now I'm volunteering at a hospital. Do you think helping at a research lab will help my chances of getting in, or do you think volunteering is enough?"

On and on he went. Every question was some variation of *how do I get into medical school?*

Finally, I interrupted the young student: "Look, I get it. You're focused on getting into medical school right now. But don't you have any questions about what med school is actually like? Aren't you curious about what awaits you once you start medical school, choose your specialty, apply to residency, and become a real, practicing physician? How do you know being a doctor is actually a good fit for you? What other career options have you considered?"

He paused and looked at me like a deer in headlights. Finally, he responded: "Yeah, I do wonder about those things. But to be honest . . . I don't even know where to begin. Getting into medical school is such a tall hurdle that it's tough to see past that sometimes. It's hard enough to figure out what I need to do to get in—much less what happens after that. I don't know any doctors personally, and real information about what it's *really* like to become a doctor is hard to come by."

He paused again, cleared his throat, and asked me, "So . . . what is med school really like?"

And that's when the idea to write this book first hit me.

There were enough books, internet forums, and seminars about *how* to get into medical school. Pre-meds have been devouring such information for decades, even more so as getting into medical school becomes increasingly competitive.

I decided to instead write a book that frankly describes *what it's like* getting into medical school—and beyond. I would write an exposé about being a medical student, a resident, a fellow, and a brand-new attending physician—all from the perspective of someone fresh out of the process.

They say you should always know your audience when writing. This book is written first and foremost for those brave souls immersed in the continuum of medical education. This is for pre-meds who are still trying to decide if med school is for them, as well as those already in the process of applying to medical schools, anxious to learn more about what awaits them. This is also for the young medical student just starting his or her journey, a guide for what to expect and how to navigate the sometimes murky waters of med school and residency. Finally, this is for the seasoned medical student, resident, fellow, or fresh attending who wants to commiserate or borrow experiences and advice from someone else in their shoes. (*Attending* is one term for a physician who is done with training—a bona fide doctor, with all the status and remuneration expected with that position.)

Of course, all readers are welcome. I hope this book will be enlightening to friends and family of young doctors-to-be, nostalgic for practicing or retired physicians, or at least entertaining to the curious general public. To ensure a variety of opinions and viewpoints, I've included stories and advice from over a dozen other young physicians from medical schools and residency programs throughout the country. Most contributors were gracious enough to provide their real names; others (whose pseudonyms appear in quotation marks) preferred to remain anonymous.

PART I

THE PREMEDICAL YEARS

1.
WHY GO TO MED SCHOOL?

Time for Some Soul Searching

For the pre-meds reading this book, the first thing you need to figure out is *why* you are a pre-med. *Why do you want to go to med school and become a doctor?*

The entire admissions process will run much more smoothly if you take time up front to examine your thoughts and motivations. You should compile four or five of your top reasons to become a physician. Once you have that solidified, everything else falls into place, including your admissions essays and interviews. It's also critical to have those reasons to fall back on when you're exhausted from studying, suffering academic or personal setbacks, or wondering why in the hell you're doing all of this. Having a clear sense of purpose can be invaluable before, during, and after medical school.

A few dozen reasons pop up with regularity. Some are better than others. And some seem great from the pre-med perspective and become less appealing or even irrelevant once one actually enters medical practice. In this chapter, I subject the most commonly cited reasons for becoming a doctor to a reality check—through the lens of a young, private practice physician fresh out from the decade-long slog of medical training. As with everything in this book, I encourage you to take my commentary with a grain of salt and speak with as many other physicians as you can find to round out your view.

And now, it's time to crush some youthful optimism . . .

1. I WANT TO HELP PEOPLE.

This is the number one most commonly stated reason for wanting to go into medicine. Interestingly, I *didn't* include it in my own application essays or bring it up in my interview. Not that I don't enjoy helping people in my work today. But personally, this reason alone would never have been enough for me to consider going through everything necessary to become a physician.

After all, plenty of occupations help people. The young girl working in the Target aisles can help you find a can of beans. Police officers help people out of scary situations every day. Firefighters risk life and limb to help people save their belongings and lives. Crossing guards help children safely cross the street. You get the idea.

I wouldn't dissuade anyone from considering a career in medicine based on the motivation of wanting to help people—far from it. This desire to help might be the one thing that keeps you sane when you're in the county ER at midnight and attempt to perform a physical exam on a belligerent, drunk homeless man who cusses you out, spits on your shoes, and tells you to leave him the hell alone and that he only came into the ER because it's −20°F outside and he had been kicked out of all the shelters. (Yes, some variant of this encounter *will* happen to you more than once in your training.)

Even as a practicing physician, there will be times when everything annoys you. Your board recertification will be due, along with its outrageous fees. A hospital administrator will bug you about your incomplete documentation. A nurse will submit an anonymous report that you were short with her after your long overnight call. There will be days where you wonder why you went through everything you did.

And then, when everything seems to be encouraging you to take an early retirement, some patient you treated several weeks ago and had nearly forgotten will spot you in the hall and say, "Doctor! Thank you so much for everything you did! Our daughter just got discharged from the NICU yesterday. My wife was petrified when they told her she needed an emergency C-section, but you really put her at ease and helped her through it all."

In virtually every field of medicine, you will help patients in direct and meaningful ways that people in most professions will never experience. So there's nothing wrong with wanting to go into medicine for this reason. Just realize there *are* other ways to help people, and you should probably have some other, different reasons to make the whole process worthwhile. Also, for the pre-meds reading this book, know that your admissions officer's eyes will glaze over after reading or hearing this reason for the five hundredth time this admissions cycle.

2. I LIKE SCIENCE, BIOLOGY, ANATOMY, PHYSIOLOGY, AND SO ON.

This is another very common reason people give for wanting to become a physician, and again, a very reasonable one that I think *should* be somewhere on everyone's list. After all, the entire span of premedical coursework and the countless hours of lectures and studying required throughout the four years of medical school are very directly rooted in the life sciences. Sure, you won't have to draw the Krebs cycle as a practicing physician, but you will need to be able to read a journal that references it and to understand it at a general level. In other words, a physician reads, eats, and breathes materials based on the sciences throughout his or her career. Doctors can't be science-phobes.

But similar to wanting to help people, an enjoyment of science is hardly reason enough to go through all the work and time of becoming a physician. There are *many* fields based on the sciences, including engineering, nursing, computer science, teaching and academics, materials science, and bioengineering, among others. And again, know that your admissions officer's eyes will glaze over after reading or hearing this reason for the five hundredth time this admissions cycle.

3. I WANT TO UNDERSTAND THE HUMAN BODY.

Close cousin to the preceding reason, this merits a separate entry because, of all the reasons listed here, I actually think this is the one thing that you can best accomplish by graduating from medical school and completing a residency program—regardless of specialty. With all due respect to academic experts in physiology, biochemistry, and anatomy, as well as the multitude of nonphysician health professionals who make up today's complex medical care teams, you gain a unique blend of book smarts and real-world knowledge about the big picture and tiny intricacies of the human body by spending roughly a decade of your life devoted almost fully to learning about the human body.

I would never go toe-to-toe with a biochemist about the details of ATP generation, nor would I argue with a seasoned urology physician's assistant about the best way to place a difficult urinary catheter. There are PhD researchers who know infinitely more about specific biological and chemical components of the human body. And there are health professionals—including nursing assistants, phlebotomists, perfusionists, and nurse practitioners—who have worked for years in their specific capacities and likely know those fields as well as or better than the average physician.

But in my experience, when it comes to instilling a holistic and almost intuitive understanding of the human body, few experiences come close to medical school coupled with a residency education—especially when you add at least a few years in practice. In medical school, a seasoned physician once told me, you know you're making headway when you can walk into a patient's room and within seconds know if the patient is healthy, kind of sick, or deathly ill.

Medical students are forced to memorize thousands of pieces of information, including every muscle and bone in the body, virtually all major chemical processes responsible for human life, the pharmacokinetics and pharmacodynamics of all basic drug groups used in modern medicine, and the physiologic workings of all major organ systems. Residents then work countless hours in hospitals with real patients, forced to make myriad decisions with incomplete information, sometimes after working thirty hours straight. As a board certified physician, you can't necessarily regurgitate all of those details you once memorized. But the important knowledge gleaned from the learning experience remains. Couple that with practical experience, and an experienced physician can know within seconds if a patient needs immediate attention, based on their presentation and clinical history.

4. I WANT TO WORK WITH PEOPLE AND/OR THE GENERAL PUBLIC.

I'm pretty sure I said this in my med school interviews and application essays. Prior to becoming a physician, much of my working life was spent at a computer screen. This wasn't my preference, and I realized early on that I liked working with the general public and meeting new people every day—not just the same coworkers day in and day out. It should be obvious that there are *many* jobs out there beyond medicine that could fulfill this requirement. But in general, becoming a physician will, for better or worse, meet this need for mingling with the masses, so long as one doesn't become a pathologist or radiologist.

However, many applicants to med school may not fully appreciate what working with the general public really means. It's easy to work at a trendy bar in college or some retail job in high school and think you really enjoy interacting with people all day. But depending on where you work as a physician, you really will see the entire gamut of society, much more than you do in ordinary jobs. And even if you end up in a suburban community hospital, your training in med school or residency will almost certainly expose you to segments of society that you may have previously not spent much time with.

I hate to generalize, and there are exceptions, but many middle- and upper-income folks considering going to med school have not spent a lot of time exposed to the homeless, incarcerated, drug-addicted, psychotic, and other marginalized population groups. This may be especially true for younger applicants whose only experience outside of a comfortable suburban home has been four years in a diverse but affluent college town.

I don't say any of this to disparage this reason for wanting to go to medical school. I still derive much satisfaction every day from meeting people from all walks of life and interacting with them in a very intimate and meaningful way not possible with most jobs. But do know that at some point in your medical career you will probably meet people who are unsavory, manipulative, and potentially quite dangerous. And you will still be expected to empathize with them and provide them with top-notch medical care.

5. I WANT TO WORK WITH MY HANDS AND DO TANGIBLE WORK.

This was actually a significant reason for me to consider a career in medicine, which I stated during my interviews and in my essays. I find it satisfying to spend at least part of my workday actually *doing* something with my hands, whether it be placing a central line, performing a nerve block, or even just laying hands on a patient during a physical exam. I think many applicants share this desire, particularly those attracted to the surgical or interventional fields.

Unfortunately, like every profession in our increasingly technological society, medicine will likely require a hefty amount of time at a computer screen. Federal initiatives require the use of electronic medical records, which are gradually replacing the traditional method of dictating patient notes, and require physicians to divide their time between actually interacting with patients and documenting those interactions on a computer. Worse, documentation has become increasingly synonymous with billing and reimbursement, such that half the stuff physicians are required to type into notes these days is read only by billing staff and is of little or no clinical value.

So if you're still deciding whether you want to go into medicine, or are choosing your specialty, be aware that gone are the days when a doctor just bounced from room to room chatting with patients, performing some exams, and quickly jotting down a visit note or dictating exam findings. You *will* be using an electronic medical record system at some point in your career.

I should say that this will be worst in medical school, where you will be expected to write the lengthiest and most elaborate patient notes possible, largely as a training exercise to help you organize your thoughts. It will get better in residency but will still be somewhat onerous. By the time you have finished residency, you will be able to count in the triple digits the hours of your life spent writing discharge summaries and H&P's (history and physical exams).

But for the most part, it's not horrible once you're done with training and either have residents and fellows writing all your notes as an academic attending or likely have some combination of scribes and mid-level providers helping you with your documentation in private practice. Also, this varies greatly based on specialty. Procedural specialties such as surgery, anesthesiology, and interventional medical fields tend to involve less paperwork than more diagnostic and long-term management specialties like family practice, internal medicine, and pediatrics.

6. I WANT TO MAKE A LOT OF MONEY.

Obviously it's career suicide to mention this during your med school interviews or write it in an application essay. But it's almost always a factor, unless you're independently wealthy from prior work or family money. So *do* doctors actually make a lot of money?

The answer isn't simple. In general, once done with training and working full-time, most physicians are among the top few percentages of income earners in the country. This varies from the top 5 percent to the top 1 to 2 percent, depending largely on the specialty, geographic area of practice, hours worked, and whether one is in academics or private practice. But even in the absolutely lowest-paid specialties in the lowest-paid cities in an academic or charity practice, it's a rare physician job that doesn't make six figures. And compared to the vast majority of Americans, that's nothing to sneeze at.

So you're not going to starve, and you're going to be able to live in an area with good schools and drive a nice car and vacation in nice places. Are you going to drive a $250,000 sports car, own a professional sports team, and live in one of those fancy houses in Beverly Hills perched on a mudslide-prone cliff? Probably not—unless you're clever and tenacious enough to capitalize on your medical training in some outside-the-box way. And yes, you're going to pay a lot of taxes.

In summary, I would never call medicine a "road to riches," especially when you consider that you will spend roughly a decade after college earning about the same as a fast-food manager on an hourly basis. This is doubly true if you don't have a family member or generous benefactor paying for your education, as most U.S. docs come out of training with student loans in excess of a quarter-million dollars. It's *very* difficult to get out of paying your student loans, and you will pay the equivalent of a mortgage payment each month for a decade or two to get rid of these. Finally, the typical physician has given up years of potential wealth building and compounded interest by the time she is making the big bucks.

That said, for the foreseeable future you can rest assured that a medical career will almost guarantee you a well-paid and respected job for the rest of your life. For most qualified med school applicants, however, there are likely many other careers that could also provide these things. So I don't think there's anything wrong with a qualified applicant wanting to enter a career with good earning potential. But I agree with others who caution against choosing the path of medical school *primarily* for the money. If this is your only or primary motivating factor, many times in your training and career you will struggle and wonder why you put yourself through all of this.

7. I WANT FINANCIAL STABILITY AND/OR JOB SECURITY.

This is essentially my conclusion for reason #6, and if you're going to reference money in your interviews or application essays, it should probably be worded more like this. I think this is a very reasonable base criterion to have for any career you are considering, assuming that you have the intelligence and wherewithal to enter such a profession.

I would ignore anyone who glibly responds, "You should have gone to Wall Street if you were interested in money!" Not everyone wants to work in finance, petroleum engineering, or whatever other well-paid career is in vogue at the time, but that doesn't mean you're an evil Scrooge if you feel you should be fairly rewarded for choosing a career you are interested in that requires a massive commitment of time, energy, and money on the front end.

8. I WANT A JOB THAT IS HIGHLY RESPECTED.

I didn't care much about this, but I know some people do. In retrospect, I suppose it is nice to have a career that most people view as a valuable and positively contributing profession. I'm sure it gets old always having to explain how being a tobacco executive really isn't *that* bad. And for the most part, I think society does still hold medicine in relatively high regard and that you won't be terribly disappointed if this is a reason you want to go to med school.

Do be forewarned, however, that Veteran's Administration hospitals are probably the only place you'll work where patients consistently respond with a hearty, "Whatever you say, doc!" Nowadays, patients come into clinic armed with WebMD printouts and quotes from Dr. Oz, and you will have to answer to such things regardless of their merit. Also, in a world increasingly concerned about rising health care costs and the threatened insolvency of Medicare, well-paid physicians are easy fodder for criticism from politicians, Facebook friends, and the random guy sitting next to you on the plane. Even as a clueless, powerless, and penniless med student, I was surprised by how often I received unsolicited opinions about the state of the American health care system.

9. MY RELATIVE OR FAMILY FRIEND IS A DOCTOR, SO I WANT TO BE ONE, TOO.

Probably not the strongest reason to mention to an admissions officer, but I'm sure it makes its way into more than one essay each year. If you do have a close relative or family friend who is a physician, it's certainly good to spend as much time as possible with that person. Pick her brain about how she ended up in her position, how she has enjoyed her career, and what she thinks about your reasons for wanting to go into medicine and the future of the profession.

On that note, a word of advice regarding talking to practicing doctors about the future of the profession. There are always folks in every profession who will tell you the "glory days" are long gone and you would be a fool to enter the field. Sometimes there's merit to this, but other times it's just a matter of people not liking change. This can be difficult to discern, which is why it's important to get multiple perspectives and not rely solely on one person's narrative, even if she is a close relative or friend.

10. MY PARENTS, TEACHERS, AND/OR OTHER FIGURES OF AUTHORITY WANT ME TO BE A DOCTOR.

In general, this is a *horrible* reason for becoming a doctor. The commitment during training and the rest of your working life is *way* too big to do it for somebody else. It's fine if you independently want to become a doctor *and* your parents also think you should. Just be sure your decisions are not too heavily influenced by others. Sure, you may be good at science or tie knots very well or just be really smart, but none of these are sufficient reasons to become a doctor. To quote the cinematic masterpiece *Harold & Kumar Go to White Castle*, "Just 'cause you're hung like a moose doesn't mean you gotta do porn."

11. I'M SMART AND GOOD AT SCIENCE, SO EVERYONE SAYS I SHOULD BECOME A DOCTOR.

Same response as for reason #10. Decide to become a physician for yourself, not for anybody else.

12. I WANT TO BE A SURGEON, CARDIOLOGIST, OR SOME OTHER SPECIFIC TYPE OF PHYSICIAN.

Obviously, if you want to be a pediatric cardiothoracic surgeon or some other highly specialized physician, you have to go to medical school. My only caution about this is that people rarely end up becoming exactly the type of physician they think they are going to be when they enter medical school. Half the purpose of med school is to expose future doctors to the myriad specialty choices available to them.

The years of residency training are a tremendous investment. Young physicians should have as much information about their future careers as possible before committing to a specialty. Certainly, there *were* people in my medical school class who came in saying, "I'm going to do orthopedics" and ended up doing orthopedics. But for every one of them, there are at least two or three who ended up doing something quite different from their initial plans.

Keep in mind, too, that simply getting into medical school is no guarantee you can pursue the specialty of your choice. I talk about this in greater detail later, but in short, I will say that very few premeds understand how specialty selection occurs. Even most first- and second-year med students don't understand it. It is based on many factors, including your med school academic standing, standardized test scores, research experience, and networking abilities.

Unless you scored in the top 20 percent of people taking the Medical College Admission Test (MCAT), got accepted to nearly every medical school to which you applied, and are generally an excellent test taker, socially amiable, and not completely averse to getting involved in some research projects, be very careful about pursuing a career in medicine with a specific specialty in mind. You may find out too late that you don't have what you need to get into your specialty of choice.

13. I WANT TO DO MEDICAL RESEARCH.

If you are completely committed to being a career medical scientist, look into the MD-PhD combined programs. As of now, you can get your entire medical education paid for with a modest stipend, you will have a leg up on specialty and residency selection, and it will nicely pave a path into academic medicine and a career in research. Granted, you will spend upward of twelve to sixteen years after college in some form of medical training, but this is by far the best way to pursue this type of research. Grant money is very hard to come by these days, and having both medical and research backgrounds is of great value.

14. I WANT TO PRACTICE GLOBAL MEDICINE AND VOLUNTEER ABROAD.

There are plenty of opportunities for physicians to practice abroad and pursue global public health initiatives. However, be forewarned: very few people or organizations will *pay* you for this type of work. Most physicians who go on mission trips fixing cleft palates in African babies volunteer their own time and money to do so—often to the tune of several thousand dollars of lost wages, airfare, and supplies.

15. I WANT A FLEXIBLE EDUCATION THAT WILL ALLOW ME TO WORK IN BUSINESS, TECHNOLOGY, EDUCATION, AND SO ON.

Completion of medical school *with* residency does open many doors. Some can be quite lucrative, though they're usually riskier, with less consistent payouts than traditional medical practice. However, realize that you will drive yourself crazy if you start the long process of medical education with the primary goal of doing something other than practicing medicine. Ninety percent of your training prepares you to practice medicine. You will too often wonder why you are wasting so many years of your life learning all this stuff if your primary goal is to someday become CEO of a hospital or a medical technology consultant.

16. I'VE WATCHED [INSERT MEDICAL DRAMA SHOW HERE] AND THINK BEING A DOCTOR LOOKS AWESOME.

I really hope this isn't anybody's primary reason for wanting to become a doctor. If it is, keep it to yourself during the admissions process. Nearly every medical drama is inaccurate in virtually all medical details and practicalities. These shows are "for entertainment purposes only," as they say.

One exception is *Scrubs*, which many physicians will tell you is one of the most accurate portrayals of life as a doctor that has graced the television screen in recent history—ironic since the show was written as a parody of serious medical dramas. This prime-time comedy paralleled much of my own medical training, with both the show and my time in med school ending in the spring of 2010. *Scrubs* never tried to realistically portray tense moments in the operating room, but it expertly captured the everyday struggles, fears, hopes, and joys of medical trainees. And I've yet to see another medical series so painfully accurate in its depiction of the medical hierarchy—the sacred totem pole with attending physicians at the top, from which everything bad and smelly travels downward to the fellows, residents, interns, and, finally, the lowly medical students.

17. MY FRIEND OR RELATIVE SUFFERED FROM OR DIED FROM SOME DISEASE, SO I WANT TO HELP FIND A CURE OR HELP PATIENTS WITH THIS DISEASE.

It's okay to have such a specific goal. But much like entering medicine with a very specific specialty in mind, you must acknowledge the real possibility that you will end up doing something completely different, for any number of reasons—not least of which is that the disease you wanted to cure has since been cured or is now easily treatable with new technology. Remember, a decade or more will pass from the time you commit to becoming a physician and actually finish medical training. A lot can happen in that time.

2.
GETTING INTO MED SCHOOL

Easier Said Than Done

When it comes to getting into med school, there's really no magic bullet. And sometimes the numbers game just doesn't work in your favor. For every qualified, superb med school candidate who gets accepted, there's another qualified, superb candidate rejected. I was shocked when one of the smartest and most capable medical students in my class told me his first application had been rejected. Sometimes it happens, and there's just no great explanation for it.

There are far fewer American medical school seats than there are people who want to fill them. To maximize your acceptance chances, you need to do very well in school, ideally starting in high school and certainly throughout college. You need to excel in the sciences and do very well on the MCAT. You need to think very carefully about your reasons for wanting to become a physician and prove to the admissions committee, through actions and words, that you have undertaken this self-reflection and are committed to your goals. Finally, you need to pursue activities outside of school that help convince the admissions committee you will make a good physician and you know what you're getting into. Being somehow unique and different from every other applicant never hurts either.

COMBINED UNDERGRADUATE–MEDICAL
SCHOOL PROGRAMS

If you're a precocious, overachieving high school student convinced that med school is right for you, then consider applying to one of the fifty or so medical schools that offers a combined undergraduate and medical school experience. These programs allow students to graduate with bachelor of science and doctor of medicine degrees in a mere seven years—one year less than the typical aggregate of four years for undergraduate studies and four years for medical school. Admission to these programs usually requires top-notch high school performance, demonstrated maturity and commitment to becoming a physician, and a minimum MCAT score and GPA after completion of three years of college. The application timelines for these programs are usually similar to those for ordinary four-year colleges. As always, specific requirements and due dates vary among schools. I encourage you to be *very* sure this is what you want to do before you submit your application materials. Choosing to become a physician is a monumental and difficult decision—much more so for a sixteen-year-old high school student.

COLLEGE AND MED SCHOOL PREREQUISITES

Let's say you're not Doogie Howser. Instead, you're following the more typical approach of applying to med school during or shortly after college. In that case, the fun really starts in your final years of high school when you are applying to colleges. You want to get into the best college you possibly can. You don't need to break the bank going to an elite private college—though it probably wouldn't hurt. And it's not the end of the world if you don't get into an Ivy League school. But if you're considering going to your state's flagship, public, four-year university versus a small regional college that nobody outside of a fifty-mile radius has ever heard of, my advice is to go to the better-known four-year university.

I know, with all the concerns about skyrocketing college tuition and student debt, it is becoming increasingly popular for students to go to less expensive colleges—or even attend a community college for the first two years before transferring to a larger school. I wholeheartedly agree with this logic for most students and most career paths. Unfortunately, I don't think this is good advice for pre-med students applying to med school.

For better or worse, there is still a lot of academic snobbery and elitism among med school admissions committees. A large component of your med school application is your performance on the prerequisite science courses that are usually taken during your freshman and sophomore years of college. And an A in general chemistry at Springfield Community College is not equivalent to an A in general chemistry from Harvard University, UC Berkeley, or even Wayne State University.

Most entry-level science courses that constitute the bulk of med school prerequisite coursework are heavily curved, thereby making grades largely dependent on the overall performance of the class. There will always be exceptions, but the caliber of students at a two-year community college is typically quite different from those at a large four-year university. Most students know this, and med school admissions officers definitely know it. If you earned a 4.0 GPA in all of your basic science classes at a community college, then transferred to a large four-year university and ended with an overall GPA of 3.5, most admissions committees will look at all of your grades with a jaundiced eye. They will assume that had you taken all of your classes at the four-year university, your overall GPA probably would have been 3.0.

I'm not saying you absolutely won't get into med school if you go to a small, obscure college or start at a community college and transfer to a four-year university. Nor am I saying that you're sunk if you are already in this position. But it doesn't help your chances of getting into med school. You will have to work extra hard on other parts of your med school application to convince the admissions committee you have the intellectual wherewithal to excel in medical school.

Once you're in college, you really can study whatever you want. Most incoming medical students still arrive with bachelor of science degrees in biology, chemistry, or biochemistry. But this is no longer a requirement for admission to med school. In fact, admissions committees love applicants who prove they can excel in their prerequisite science coursework while also mastering completely different and unique fields of study. For example, an applicant graduating summa cum laude with a degree in flute performance and a 3.9 GPA on her basic science coursework would be an admission officer's dream come true. On the other hand, an art history major with a B in every science class has no better chances than a biology major with a 3.0 GPA—which are pretty bad chances.

As for the "pre-med" major that many college students talk about, this isn't even an actual field of study at most colleges. It's certainly not required for admission to med school. When college students refers to themselves as a "pre-med," that really just means that they want to go to medical school after college. It doesn't necessarily describe a college major, field of study, or the student's actual chances of successfully matriculating in medical school. Anyone can call himself a pre-med. It's more a state of mind than an actual title.

Most medical schools require applicants to complete a specific set of *prerequisite* courses. Most of these are science classes, including a year each of biology, general chemistry, organic chemistry, and physics, and a semester of biochemistry. Many schools also require some exposure to calculus, statistics, anatomy, and physiology. To determine exactly which classes you need to take in college, you need to go to the website of each med school you are considering and make sure you have everything covered. You will find oddball schools with unusual requirements. So if such a school is high on your list, you need to make sure you take all of that school's prerequisite classes.

MEDICAL COLLEGE ADMISSION TEST (MCAT)

By your junior year of college, you need to think very seriously about whether you actually want to attend medical school. Reading this book is a great first step! Doing as well as you possibly can in all of your classes is the next step. According to the Association of American Medical Colleges (AAMC), the average college GPA of first-year U.S. medical students in 2016 was 3.7. Graduating with a GPA at or above this number will dramatically improve your chances of getting into medical school.

Once you commit to applying to medical school, you need to start preparing for the MCAT, a standardized, computer-based, multiple-choice exam administered at commercial testing sites throughout the country. Most medical schools in the United States and Canada require applicants to take the MCAT and submit their scores. It is considered an "equalizer" of variation in college and coursework difficulty. It is a single, standardized number that all medical schools can use when evaluating applicants, regardless of each student's college and field of study. Much like the SAT and ACT exams required for college admissions, the MCAT is the single most important exam you will take in the process of applying to medical school.

Back when I applied to medical school in 2005, the MCAT was administered twice a year. It was a pencil-and-paper exam with three multiple-choice sections and a free-response essay section. A few hundred hopeful pre-meds showed up early at a high school cafeteria. A proctor recited the rules, a starting time was announced, and everyone worked diligently for several hours. Months later, we received our scores, which ranged from 3 to 45. A score of 30 or above was the goal.

Nowadays, the exam is offered twenty times a year, with most test dates concentrated in the summer and early fall. There are now four sections: Biological and Biochemical Foundations of Living Systems; Chemical and Physical Foundations of Biological Systems; Psychological, Social, and Biological Foundations of Behavior; and Critical Analysis and Reasoning Skills. Each is scored from a low of 118 to a high of 132, with a midpoint of 125. Section scores combined create a total score ranging from 472 to 528, with a midpoint of 500. The essay section was scrapped a few years ago.

Since the new MCAT scoring system was adopted, the AAMC has published one report detailing average MCAT scores of applying and accepted U.S. medical students in 2016. According to this report, the average MCAT score of accepted students was 509, compared to an average score of 502 for all applicants. Of course, your goal is to achieve a score at or above 509.

You should start preparing for the MCAT early in your junior year. There are hundreds of books, online materials, and in-person courses you can take to help you prepare. Though the MCAT website says you don't need to take any specific college courses prior to taking the exam, common sense indicates you should probably wait until you've taken your prerequisite science classes before sitting for the MCAT. In addition to some basic statistics and reasoning questions, it's essentially a big science exam, focusing on biology, chemistry, biochemistry, physics, and behavioral sciences including psychology and sociology.

I leave it to you to determine the best way to study for this exam, except for these musts: (1) become familiar with the exam format, number of questions, and timing, and (2) explore the MCAT website and take advantage of the many available sample questions and demonstrations of the computer interface. Beyond that, I encourage you to explore the myriad available books, software, and courses. By this point in your academic career you probably know which study techniques work best for you. If not, there are hundreds of people willing to offer their opinions—for a price.

Plan on taking the MCAT sometime during the spring of your junior year. You can register for the MCAT anytime during the winter or early spring of that year. Just go to the AAMC website, enter a bunch of personal information, and pay a $300 registration fee. Yep, it's the first of many exorbitant exam fees you will pay as you travel the long, bumpy, and costly road of medical training.

As with most standardized exams you will take in your medical career, you'll spend most of a day at a commercial testing center—usually a big room with a few dozen cubicles each equipped with a computer and headphones to keep out extraneous noise. You walk in with your registration slip, photo ID, and a snack. Somebody takes your photo and possibly frisks you. You put all your belongings into a locker. Finally, you are escorted to your own private cubicle, where you will spend over six hours answering 230 multiple-choice questions on a computer.

You will receive your MCAT score roughly a month after you take it. By the time this book is in print, there will likely have been several sets of students who have taken the newly scored MCAT and gained admission to medical school. The AAMC website will likely have statistics available regarding the average MCAT scores of incoming medical students. Compare your score to the statistics, and see where you fit in the big picture.

If your application is otherwise stellar—with a solid GPA, good letters of recommendation, impressive extracurricular activities, and no red flags—you're probably good to go as long as your MCAT score is in the general ballpark of the average score of previously accepted applicants. However, if your score is lower than you'd like and the rest of your application is fairly average among people applying to medical school, then you may consider retaking the MCAT.

Thankfully, you can take the exam up to three times per year, so you can spend a few months better preparing for the exam and take it again in the late spring or summer. Depending on the school, admissions committees will use either your highest score or an average of all your submitted MCAT scores. You should register for your second exam as soon as you decide you want to retake it, as exam dates fill up quickly as the year progresses.

LETTERS OF RECOMMENDATION

Toward the end of your junior year, you should contact trusted faculty and mentors and ask them to write you positive letters of recommendation for your application. Note the adjective "positive." You should also specify *positive* letters of recommendation from your faculty. If you sense any hesitation in response to your request, keep looking. I know this seems like a burdensome task to ask of people, but your faculty are accustomed to such requests. Writing letters of recommendation goes with being a professor, and they inevitably have some boilerplate letters on file that they can quickly modify to fit your profile and career goals.

Medical schools require varying numbers of letters of recommendation, but three is a pretty standard minimum. You should find at least two science faculty members to write letters on your behalf, and if possible at least one letter from a research adviser or mentor who knows you very well. You can always ask department chairs or other academic "big names" for letters, but it's generally better to have a well-written, personalized letter from someone who actually knows you and can honestly speak to your strengths. Avoid asking teaching assistants for letters. It never hurts to give specific deadlines to your letter writers. Finally, you should ask for one more letter than you actually need, in case someone unexpectedly doesn't deliver at the last minute.

PERSONAL STATEMENT

Around the same time, you should start thinking about your application essay, also called the *personal statement*. Like everything else in the admissions process, there are dozens of books on how to write a winning application essay. You can buy packets of sample "accepted" essays. You can even pay people to review and edit your essays. If writing isn't your strong suit, then you may feel the need to solicit some of these services. But ultimately, admissions officers are really looking for three basic things from your application essay.

First, they want to know whether you can string two sentences together in a coherent fashion. This is the easy part. Again, if you weren't blessed with literary talents, enlist the help of friends, family, or faculty to review your essay. Many college campuses offer essay review services. There are also for-profit services online.

Second, admissions officers want to see a glimmer of who you are behind the GPA, MCAT score, academic awards, and extracurricular activities. Be honest. Share a personal story or experience. Show them who you are as a person.

Finally, they want to know without a doubt that you have really thought long and hard about your decision to become a doctor. This is the most important part. Your application essay should easily unfold once you've clearly identified *why* you want to be a physician. If you're still struggling with this, I encourage you to reread the previous chapter and compare your thoughts to the many common reasons people state for becoming physicians. Your primary goal should be to convey to the admissions committee what is driving you to become a physician—why you want to go through the many years of intense study, long hours, and personal sacrifice. You must demonstrate that you understand the many challenges ahead of you and know full well what you're getting into.

MED SCHOOL APPLICATION

During the summer between your junior and senior years, you need to revisit the AAMC website and register for the American Medical College Application Service (AMCAS), a centralized system that allows you to submit all of your application materials to one place. An online interface is used to electronically upload your demographic information, academic history, work experience, transcripts, reference contacts, and personal statement. Of course, there is a fee. As of 2017, it costs $160 to register for AMCAS and submit your materials to one medical school. Each additional school is an extra $38. Fee assistance is available if you qualify.

A perennial question among pre-meds is how many medical schools to apply to. According to the AAMC, 53,042 med school applicants submitted an astounding total of 830,016 applications in 2017. Simple math produces an average of just under sixteen applications per applicant. That isn't necessarily the correct answer to the perennial question, but it's probably a good place to start. Sending your application materials to sixteen schools using AMCAS will cost you at least $730, which isn't chump change.

If your application materials, MCAT score, and GPA are in line with the average numbers of accepted med school applicants, then applying to around a dozen med schools is probably more than enough. It's not worth the extra money to apply to more. Choose some areas of the country you wouldn't mind living in for four years, do your research, and pick a dozen of your favorite med schools. Try to pick a few "reach" schools with academic numbers a bit stronger than yours and a couple of "safety" schools, and *always* include your home state's public school, assuming you have one. You almost always will receive a warmer welcome at your own state school, and lower in-state tuition can save you tens of thousands of dollars.

Some schools expressly state on their websites and on the AAMC website that they *do not accept any out-of-state applicants*. According to publicly available reports on the AAMC website, in 2016 there were six schools that did not accept a single out-of-state applicant, and a total of 1,184 out-of-state students applied to those six schools combined. That's thousands of dollars in application fees down the drain. Even more schools are notorious about accepting only a very small fraction of their applicants from out of state. These things change from year to year, so do your research before you add a school to your AMCAS application list.

Some medical schools offer an Early Decision Program (EDP). The deadline is usually sometime in early August. If you're entirely committed to one first-choice medical school and are ready to submit your application by this early date, you may have slightly better chances of being accepted in the EDP. The idea is that med schools would prefer to have some good, committed applicants locked in early in the process, reducing the number of applicants they have to review and interview later in the year during the normal admissions cycle. Of course, if your application is well below the standard of accepted medical students at that school, applying in the EDP is unlikely to help you.

The AMCAS application you submit online is called your *primary application*. During the fall of your senior year, you will hopefully receive requests from medical schools for *secondary applications*. Sound like more work? It is—but this is a good thing. If a medical school you applied to sends you a secondary application, it means you met that school's baseline requirements for GPA and MCAT scores. In sum, you made the short list, and they want to know more about you.

Secondary applications are traditionally paper-based, but they are increasingly completed online in a format similar to the AMCAS. They usually ask a few extra questions about why you want to study medicine in that part of the country or if you have any specific ties to that medical school. They almost always require yet another essay or two, often with specific questions that you must address. And, of course, they without fail ask for *more money*. Secondary application fees are typically $20 to $40, but some are as high as $100. Unfortunately, a few schools are notorious about sending virtually everyone who applies to them a secondary application, only to reject the applicants within days of receiving a completed (and paid for) secondary application.

When completing secondary application essays, the same general rules apply. Be honest, be coherent, and be clear that you know what you are doing, why you are doing it, and what you are in for. Try to include some honest reasons why you are interested in the specific med school or location. Whatever you do, be careful not to inadvertently send the secondary application essay you so eloquently wrote for School A to School B!

As you patiently wait for the secondary applications to roll in, make sure your application is otherwise complete. Specifically, check your AMCAS account to make sure all your letters of recommendation are in. College faculty are notorious for dragging their feet when it comes to getting letters of recommendation uploaded. Hey, I said they are accustomed to receiving such requests; I didn't say they were good about meeting the deadlines. Send a gentle reminder by email or in person; no professor is going to intentionally give you a bad letter because you politely reminded him or her of an approaching deadline.

INTERVIEWS

Once you've returned a few secondary applications, you should hear back from schools within a few weeks. Hopefully you will get some interview offers! Med schools typically offer a few possible interview dates. The tricky part is arranging interviews around your college or work schedule. This is even trickier if you are interviewing at many schools that require air travel and overnight stays.

Of course, interviewing at faraway schools adds additional costs to an already expensive process. Once you're an attending physician, interviewing groups and hospitals will typically pay for hotels and travel. Residency and fellowship applicants sometimes also get that privilege. Unfortunately, med school applicants never get such luxuries. When it comes to travel and lodging, you're on your own, kid.

If you are applying to medical school right out of college without any prior professional experience, the med school interview might be your first-ever formal interview. Interview day can be intimidating, but at this point admissions committees are just trying to get to know you better and make sure there aren't any glaring red flags. If they're taking the time to interview you, you've already surpassed their numbers cut-offs and met their basic criteria for acceptance. Now they just want to make sure you're normal, professional, respond well to some challenging questions, and can speak intelligently about your stated research, volunteer experiences, and prior work or educational endeavors. Now is the time you're going to kick yourself for saying you're fluent in Mandarin when you only know five phrases you learned from fortune cookies.

As with everything else in the admissions process, there are dozens of books that will teach you everything you need to know about how to master the interview and win those acceptance letters. There are online resources with sample interview questions and forums where pre-med students share questions they got from various schools with which they interviewed. You're probably going to psych yourself out more than anything if you worry too much about the interview process. If you're not a natural extrovert and the idea of having a conversation with someone makes you sweat, then you should practice some mock interviews with friends, family, and advisers. If you can find someone who has already completed some interviews, so much the better.

Med school interviews are really quite simple. Buy a nice, conservative suit with neutral colors. Maintain a normal hair color and style. Arrive on time, clean and alert. Be yourself. Answer questions honestly and use the interviewers' questions as an opportunity to talk about yourself and your experiences. Ask questions if you have them, but don't go overboard just to impress people. Most important, show the admissions officers that you know why you want to become a physician and why you would like to attend their school, and that you know what you're getting into. A quick email or note thanking your interviewers afterward probably isn't necessary, but it won't hurt either.

ACCEPTED, REJECTED, OR WAIT LISTED

By late fall through early spring of your senior year, medical schools will start contacting applicants to let them know if they are accepted, rejected, or put on the dreaded *wait list*. If you are accepted to a medical school, congratulations! Most schools will give you a few weeks to think about the offer and give them an answer. The tricky part is if you're waiting on a response from another school that you liked better. You can accept a position at one school and then change your mind if you later receive a better offer. That's precisely how applicants placed on the wait list move up the list and ultimately are accepted.

Most medical schools use a *rolling admissions policy*. This means that once the AMCAS application cycle begins, schools review applications, distribute secondary applications, offer interviews, and grant admissions in a first-come, first-served manner. As their spots fill up and applicants accept offered positions, the school will likely become increasingly hesitant to offer many additional interviews. And once all spots are filled, any remaining applicants worthy of acceptance are placed on the wait list. So when it comes to submitting your AMCAS primary application, *earlier is better*!

ANOTHER DOC'S SHOES: DRESS FOR SUCCESS

As a former medical school class president and chief resident, I have always enjoyed shaping future generations of doctors. This led to my participation on the medical school interview committee and residency admissions committee. I would like to share a few tips as you're preparing for interview season. Some may seem self-explanatory, but I mention them because some medical school and residency applicants I've met in the past two years have violated each of these guidelines.

- Keep your interview outfit simple and classic. It's better to be overdressed than underdressed. Men should wear a matching suit. Women are encouraged to wear a suit with either pants or a knee-length skirt. Shirts and blouses should be neatly ironed (and no cleavage showing). Nails should be clean and well maintained. Women, if you're wearing heels, make sure they're comfortable. You'll be doing a lot of walking. Tattoos should be covered up. Take out facial piercing jewelry if possible.

- Bring a leather portfolio or similar organizer so you can take notes, keep papers, and collect business cards. Women, a purse can be a substitute for a portfolio.

- Avoid perfume or cologne; if you insist, keep it light.

- Attend the residency or medical school interview dinners that are often offered the evening before the interview. This is the best opportunity to ask residents questions informally and for residents to get to know you (and advocate for you). Having one glass of wine, one beer, or one cocktail is socially acceptable. Do not drink more than that or we'll judge you. If you're waiting at the bar for the rest of the applicants to arrive, sip on water or soda rather than an alcoholic drink. I recommend business casual attire for interview dinners.

- During your interview, be truthful. Don't make things up. The truth always comes out.

- Interviewers can (and will) look you up on social media. Make sure your Facebook, Instagram, blog, online dating profile, and so on are all appropriate (or open only to friends) prior to and during interview season.

- If you've had a criminal offense (such as consumption as a minor or DUI), be prepared to talk about it during the interview. You don't need to bring it up unless asked, but the best approach is to acknowledge your mistake and tell the interviewer what you've learned from the situation (and, if possible, find a silver lining).

- During interviews, talk at a normal pace and make good (but not intense) eye contact with the interviewer. Try a practice interview with a friend or family member to see if you have any fixable bad habits, such as peppering your sentences with "like" or "um."

- Common interview topics include your personal statement, research experience, volunteer experience, work experience, current world events, the last book you've read, a time when you worked in a group (what went well, what didn't), your strengths and weaknesses, and an obstacle you overcame.

- Always write a thank-you note to each of your interviewers as well as the program coordinator (if applicable). Handwritten notes are superior to emails, but emails are better than nothing. Write thank-you notes within a week so you remain fresh in your interviewer's mind.

- As interview season progresses, stay in touch with your program of choice. If that program is your first-choice program (or even in your top three), let the program know that. Selecting medical students and residents is somewhat like dating; we want to date (accept) someone who is really into us too. Similarly, if you've decided a program is no longer of interest to you, please let them know so they can focus on other applicants.

- Keep calm. The people involved in the interview process are generally good people with a genuine interest in shaping future generations of doctors. Most of them were in your shoes once, and we know some degree of nervousness is completely normal. Take a few deep breaths before each interview and you'll do great.

P.J. SIMONE, M.D.
MEDICAL SCHOOL AND RESIDENCY: University of Minnesota, Minneapolis

AMCAS rules dictate that by the end of April, applicants should be holding only one accepted position. This opens up any additional positions to applicants who were previously placed on wait lists. Over the next few months, medical schools continue to go down their wait lists to fill any remaining available spots. Applicants may find out they have been offered a position all the way into the first week or so of med school.

BACKUP PLANS AND SELF-ASSESSMENT

What if the summer passes and you're never offered a position at any of the medical schools to which you applied? Well, you're in good company, at least. According to the AAMC, the number of unique medical school applicants using AMCAS reached an all-time high of 52,550 in 2015. Compared to the previous year, first-time applicants increased by 4.8 percent, to 38,460. Even more applications were submitted to osteopathic (D.O.) medical schools through their own application service (called AACOMAS), and yet more were submitted to Caribbean medical schools. Only 20,630 of the 52,550 applicants— just under 40 percent—matriculated in U.S. allopathic (M.D.) medical schools in 2015.

I'll say it again: sometimes it's just a numbers game. For every qualified, superb med school candidate accepted, there's another qualified, superb candidate rejected. When it comes to your postmortem game plan, you must figure out if you really are one of the qualified, superb candidates who simply fell through the cracks and didn't make it in this round, but have a damn good chance of making it in the next round. This requires brutal honesty, introspection, and self-assessment. The alternative, of course, is that your qualifications simply were not comparable to those of applicants who got in.

ANOTHER DOC'S SHOES: HURRY UP AND WAIT!

Being put on the wait list can feel like a giant step backward after interviewing at your dream medical school. But it's not a rejection, so not all hope is lost! I applied to twelve schools, interviewed at four, was rejected by two, put on the wait list at two . . . and ultimately accepted at one. Thankfully, that's all it takes!

During my interview at the school I eventually attended, I was explicitly told that the class roster had already been filled and that I was only interviewing for a spot on the wait list. Both my interviewers told me had I interviewed earlier, I would have been accepted. So remember, with rolling admissions, it's important to attend the earliest possible interview date!

After learning I was in the top quartile on the wait list, I wrote a letter to the admissions committee and expressed my interest in the program. I believe the letter helped, and my communication continued with the admissions committee throughout the spring. June passed, and still I heard nothing. By mid-July, I was sure I was going to have to apply to med school again. Finally, the last week of July, I was off the wait list and officially accepted to med school! I moved halfway across the country and started medical school two weeks later.

DEREK DE VRY, M.D.
MEDICAL SCHOOL, RESIDENCY, AND FELLOWSHIP: Medical College of Wisconsin, Milwaukee

In the next chapter, I describe some of the options available to applicants who do not get accepted to mainstream, allopathic medical schools. The two primary alternatives are osteopathic (D.O.) schools and Caribbean medical schools. The former are increasingly becoming more like mainstream allopathic programs; the latter are quite a different story. Caribbean med schools frequently advertise themselves as "second-chance med schools" for people who can't gain acceptance to American medical schools. I encourage you to read the next chapter carefully if you find yourself in this position.

Many popular books, websites, live courses, and online forums describe the medical school admissions process as a game to be played and manipulated, with the goal of acceptance at all costs. People will teach you how to crack the code of the MCAT, write the perfect application essay, and tell interviewers exactly what they want to hear.

I have no problem with studying materials to make yourself more familiar with standardized exams or with reading sample application essays to stoke your own creative fires to write a masterful med school personal statement. But I vehemently disagree with the idea that the medical school application process is some sort of maze with a trap door, and you just need to figure out how to trick the system and fool the admissions officers to let you in that door.

It just doesn't work that way. There's one thing I'll repeat a few times by the end of the book: *Getting in is not the hardest part of medical school!* "The hardest part is getting in" is a load of bullshit that has been fed to med school applicants for the longest time. I think it's not true, and I think it's a disservice to pre-med hopefuls to perpetuate this myth.

That said, if you are in the midst of your science prerequisites in college and are finding it difficult to consistently maintain better than a 3.0 GPA, you need to think twice about whether med school is right for you. If you've taken the MCAT twice and cannot score higher than the 50th percentile, again, you need to think even harder. If you've applied to a dozen or more medical schools in two or more years and still haven't been accepted or even placed on a wait list, well, the answer seems clear.

All the crap that you have to do to get into medical school—the countless tests, science classes, standardized exams—is the *same crap* you have to do throughout the entire medical training process. That's four years of med school, during which the average student takes hundreds of exams and at least a dozen standardized exams, several of which are longer than the MCAT. That's three to seven years of residency, during which you are still memorizing gobs of material and taking standardized exams, only now with virtually no free time or consistent sleep. Then once you're done with residency, there are your specialty boards, which are of course even more standardized exams.

My point is that if you really found it extraordinarily difficult to get into medical school—after multiple attempts to rule out the "numbers game" possibility—and you were then able to somehow "fool" an admissions committee into letting you slip through the cracks, the only person you would be hurting is yourself. At worst, you might have trouble even finishing med school, in which case you would be forever saddled with significant student debt and have nothing to show for it. At best, you would likely struggle through your entire four years of med school, always at the bottom of your class, marginally passing your board exams, and with only a handful of specialty and residency locations available to you because of your poor academic performance.

If you still think you have what it takes to get into med school, this brief rundown should at least get you started in the right direction. The process can seem lengthy and convoluted. You have to register for AMCAS, write your personal statement, secure letters of recommendation, submit primary and secondary applications, and hopefully attend some interviews. But gaining acceptance to medical school really boils down to a few fundamentals. First, work hard and excel in all of your academic pursuits, especially in the sciences. Second, prepare for and do well on the MCAT. Finally, convince at least one admissions committee that you have a solid understanding of why you want to become a physician, what that means for your future, and what challenges and sacrifices you will face in your chosen career.

Oh, and don't try to stand out on the interview day by wearing a Hawaiian shirt.

3.

MED SCHOOL FLAVORS

M.D., D.O., and Caribbean

To practice medicine in the United States, you need to complete an American residency program. This is true even if you have already graduated from medical school, completed residency, and practiced medicine in another country. There are a *few* exceptions to this rule, but they are so uncommon I won't address them here.

Before applying to American residency programs, you need to have a medical degree, earned in either the United States or another country. I know most readers of this book are from the United States and are interested in attending American medical schools. But allow me to first talk about physicians who earned their medical degrees outside the United States. These folks are often called *international medical graduates* (IMGs) or *foreign medical graduates* (FMGs). With that discussion out of the way, I can then spend the remainder of the chapter focusing on the pathways available to American pre-meds.

INTERNATIONAL MEDICAL GRADUATES (IMG)

Starting about fifty years ago, the United States faced a doctor shortage — real or imagined — and looked overseas for its medical talent, particularly to India, Pakistan, and parts of East Asia and the former USSR. These IMGs often find greater financial, clinical, and research opportunities in rich countries like the United States than in their home countries.

As a result, thousands of IMGs have completed American residency programs over the last several decades—and continue to do so today. In some cases, these are experienced physicians who already have many years of practice under their belts.

More recently, there has been a push to further expand the number of physicians in the United States, to meet the needs of a rapidly increasing elderly population and expansion of health care by way of the Affordable Care Act. The problem is that most every effort to facilitate this goal has only expanded the number of medical schools in the United States. The number of residency spots has been stagnant, as they are largely dependent upon funding from Medicare sources, which has also been stagnant. So there are more American M.D. and D.O. graduates competing for the same number of residency slots, meaning even worse competition among foreign medical graduates.

OPTIONS FOR AMERICAN PRE-MEDS

If you are an American citizen and want to practice medicine in the United States, your three primary routes are an American M.D. (doctor of medicine) school, an American D.O. (doctor of osteopathic medicine) school, or a Caribbean M.D. school. I do know of a few Americans who went to more exotic locations for medical training, such as Ireland and Poland, but these options are much rarer and usually involve people who have dual citizenship or other special ties to these countries.

I'm going to do my best to objectively explain these three main pathways for American citizens to practice medicine in the United States, based on my own observations and conversations with colleagues. I'll start off by saying I know superb physicians from M.D., D.O., and Caribbean M.D. programs. Quite frankly, the competition is so fierce for American residency spots that most of the Caribbean graduates who make it to the point of practicing medicine in the United States are among the best of the best who go there for med school.

ALLOPATHIC (M.D.) AND OSTEOPATHIC (D.O.) MEDICAL SCHOOLS

When most Americans think of medical school, they picture an *allopathic* M.D. program. These schools are based on the concept of using drugs and treatments (*allo* meaning *from outside* the human body) to treat disease and suffering. Most American medical schools fall into this camp, and the foundations of the science-based form of medical training and practice we use in the United States today was established in these programs. These early pioneers (Johns Hopkins, Harvard, and the like) aimed to graduate physicians who used the scientific method in their diagnostic and treatment methods, as opposed to practicing medicine with unproven home remedies and anecdotal treatments, as was commonplace at the time. These allopathic medical schools are still the dominant force in American medicine, and the vast majority of academic chairs and bigwigs come from this background. Graduates from these schools receive an M.D. degree.

Physicians with D.O. after their names are graduates of osteopathic medical schools, which are rooted in the teachings of a nineteenth-century physician named Dr. Andrew Still. He believed most disease and suffering was related to misalignments and malfunctioning of the musculoskeletal system (*osteo* meaning *bones*). He also believed the human body contained all that was necessary to heal itself if manipulated properly, which led to the osteopathic schools having more of a homeopathic (*homeo* meaning *self*) tradition, as well as development of the osteopathic manipulation method (dubbed "OMM" by osteopaths).

These two schools of thought coexisted in the United States for over a century. Osteopathic programs have traditionally had more of a foothold in states surrounding the first program in Missouri, but they are now found worldwide.

More Similar Than Different

By the middle of the twentieth century, medicine had become increasingly organized in the United States. Professional medical societies such as the American Medical Association and the American Osteopathic Association had grown in numbers and funding. The science and therapies of medicine had become more technologically advanced and expensive. Finally, the passing of Medicare in 1965 solidified the power of the federal government and by proxy private insurance companies to establish standards of medical care using the power of reimbursement. Medical organizations clamored to have their practice techniques adopted as the standard of practice, which would be reimbursed by third-party payers.

Since that time, allopathic and osteopathic schools have come to look much more like each other, both embodying what most today would describe as "mainstream medicine." Most D.O. schools still have portions of their curriculum dedicated to the osteopathic manipulation method, but it is no longer a central component of any D.O. curriculum, and most graduates rarely or never use the OMM techniques once in practice.

There are currently separate licensing exams and residency programs for M.D. and D.O. graduates, but the number of D.O. residency programs is much smaller. Historically, many D.O. graduates have gone to M.D. residency programs, which are under the auspices of the Accreditation Council for Graduate Medical Education (ACGME) versus the American Osteopathic Association (AOA). To my knowledge, M.D. graduates can apply for and attend osteopathic residencies, but I do not personally know of any examples. Typically, D.O. students who are interested in both sets of residencies have to take both licensing exams: the United States Medical Licensing Exam (USMLE) and the Comprehensive Osteopathic Medical Licensing Examination of the United States (COMLEX-USA), as the latter is used for admissions purposes only by osteopathic residency programs.

This all may change in the years following this book's publication, a sign of even greater similarity between M.D. and D.O. programs. In February 2014, the ACGME and AOA announced that over a five-year period to end sometime around 2020, AOA-accredited residency programs will transition to ACGME recognition and accreditation. Both M.D. and D.O. graduates will have access to all residency programs. And while it may seem like this is a complete absorption of osteopathic schools into the allopathic fold, the press release does state that the D.O.-focused residency programs will still have standards of osteopathic-specific teachings, presumably including some of the OMM techniques. If nothing else, this should make the exam burden and paperwork much less onerous for osteopathic graduates.

M.D. Versus D.O.

The question remains, does it matter if one goes to an American M.D. or D.O. program?

The short answer is that for most people who just want to go out and practice in a community setting in all but the most competitive specialties (more on that later), I don't think it matters if you go to an M.D. or a D.O. program. There are great osteopathic physicians in almost all specialties in private practice settings around the country, and I can't imagine too many instances of one being denied a job because they went to a recognized D.O. school and residency. The only caveat is that there may be some reluctance from patients to use the services of osteopathic graduates in parts of the country where they are less common.

That said, if your goal is to enter into one of the most competitive specialties, such as dermatology, radiation oncology, or plastic surgery, I would say do everything you can to remove any reasons residency program directors can find to give one of these limited spots to a different candidate. For better or worse, there is still a slight bias against osteopathic programs among some academic physicians, with whom you may be dealing when trying to gain acceptance to residency programs.

I have had honest discussions with many graduates of osteopathic medical schools. A few have shared with me their passion for the osteopathic teachings, their desires for a more holistic curriculum, or how they were inspired by one of their favorite physicians growing up, who had the initials D.O. after his name instead of the more familiar M.D. But for every one of those stories, I've heard at least two or three more pragmatic reasons, along the lines of "I applied to a dozen schools, including a couple of D.O. programs that were near my state. I didn't get into any of the M.D. programs, but I got into one of the D.O. schools, and I've been pretty happy with it."

If you do go to a D.O. program, even if it is the most competitive and rigorous school in existence, you need to be prepared for at least some physicians you encounter for the rest of your life having an unspoken assumption that you went to a D.O. program because you didn't get into the more "mainstream" M.D. schools. This may be even truer in parts of the country where D.O. programs have a less established history. I'm not saying this assumption is justified or warranted, but I do think it's the reality.

CARIBBEAN M.D. PROGRAMS

If graduating from an American osteopathic school produces unspoken assumptions from some, then graduating from a Caribbean allopathic school will produce *spoken* assumptions from almost everyone. In short, I doubt you will find a single practicing physician who can honestly say they preferentially went to a Caribbean medical school while having the option to go to an American M.D. or D.O. program. If one does honestly make such a claim, then I would argue he was horribly misinformed when he made this decision.

I know many people who went to some of the better-known Caribbean medical schools, and again, some of them are among the best physicians I know. Those who soldier through and make it to the point of actually being accepted to a good American residency program usually are among the best and brightest at their schools.

The problem is, only a fraction of students who matriculate at Caribbean medical schools actually graduate—and even fewer are able to match into their top-choice specialties and residency programs.

Unlike American M.D. and D.O. programs, which have a limited number of spots available and can be selective about whom they accept into their programs, Caribbean schools are for-profit businesses that will accept virtually anyone who can at least complete an MCAT exam and pay for the school—or acquire the necessary student loans to pay.

And of course, you don't get to attend a welcoming medical school in a tropical paradise for free. Caribbean schools are all private and are frequently more expensive than their American counterparts. But the biggest drag is that simply being accepted to and matriculating at a Caribbean medical school does not guarantee that you will graduate or pass the U.S. medical boards (USMLE). Unfortunately, most students don't realize this until one, two, or even three semesters deep into their Caribbean educations, by which point they have already accumulated tens of thousands of dollars of medical school debt.

The students who do make it to American residency programs tend to have one thing in common: stellar USMLE scores, particularly on the Step 1 exam (more on that later). This is in part because most of the Caribbean schools focus heavily on preparing students for the USMLE, frequently incorporating specific board preparation classes into their curricula. They often administer a periodic practice USMLE, requiring a minimum score for advancement to the next academic level. Many students whose MCAT scores and undergraduate GPAs are well below the averages of matriculating American medical students enroll in Caribbean medical schools, only to miss the minimum required USMLE scores multiple times and ultimately dropping out, with huge student debts.

To summarize, Caribbean medical schools often advertise themselves as "second-chance medical schools," designed for dedicated American undergraduates with aspirations to medical school who, for whatever reasons, are unable to gain acceptance to traditional American M.D. or D.O. programs. There are certainly many examples of students with medical ambitions with the intellectual ability to excel in medical school who for some reason had one or two bad semesters that dropped their GPAs below the acceptable level to be accepted to an American medical school. Perhaps there was too much partying during the freshman year. Or maybe grades slipped after a loss in the family. And sometimes these students are roundly rejected by every American school to which they apply but then go on to do great things as a physician.

However, I would strongly caution students who consistently fell below the average GPAs and MCAT scores of matriculating American medical students throughout their entire undergraduate careers. Even if you are accepted to a Caribbean medical school (which is very likely if you can secure the funds and at least finish the MCAT with some semireasonable score), you are unlikely to excel on the USMLE Step 1 exam; this means it will be hard to gain acceptance to an American residency program, especially if you desire to practice in a specialty that is at all competitive. In fact, you may well not even complete four years in a Caribbean medical school. This may be the time to realize you just don't have the academic abilities required to succeed in medical school.

I say this not to be vindictive or to dash hopes. It's good to dream big. But there must be a reality check at some point. I've explained that the bottleneck to becoming an American doctor is increasingly the number of residency spots, not of medical school positions. As such, an increasing number of American residency positions are being filled by American medical graduates, who are almost invariably favored over international medical graduates (IMGs), especially those from Caribbean schools. So unless you are extremely confident that you can memorize large amounts of information and are very good at standardized exams, both of which are required to score very well on the USMLE, think long and hard about applying to Caribbean medical schools.

ANOTHER DOC'S SHOES: MED STUDENTS OF THE CARIBBEAN

Attending a Caribbean medical school is almost nobody's first choice when considering medical training options. If they say it was, either they had a friend or family member who attended one, or they are lying. This doesn't mean it is a bad option. For many people who just don't have the GPA or MCAT scores to be accepted into a U.S. medical school, the Caribbean option is a life raft— the last resort for those desperately trying to keep their head above water in the struggle to become a doctor. Caribbean medical schools have significantly lower admission standards compared with U.S. medical schools but much higher retention standards. In other words, they accept a lot of students, take their initial tuition money, and fail them if they can't stay afloat. For those who are able to figure it out and rededicate themselves to academics, this life raft can be lifesaving.

My story is like that of many other Caribbean medical school graduates. I did extremely well in high school with very little effort and never really learned how to study or be a student. I applied the same effort in college, assuming it would be enough. By my junior year, I realized I needed to work harder—but I never recovered from the initial hit to my GPA.

Dominica is in many ways an ideal place to study medicine. Being removed from family, friends, movie theaters, and a dependable power grid left me with little to do but study. So I studied—a lot. I graduated with a 3.99 GPA (that darn trauma rotation!) and scored in the 99th percentile on my board exams. This put me back on par with applicants coming out of U.S. medical schools, and I was able to match into my top-ranked anesthesiology residency. After completing a pediatric anesthesiology fellowship, I now work with some of the brightest minds in the world at St. Jude Children's Research Hospital.

KYLE MORGAN, M.D.
MEDICAL SCHOOL: Ross University School of Medicine, Portsmouth, Dominica
RESIDENCY: Medical College of Wisconsin, Milwaukee
FELLOWSHIP: Children's Hospital of Wisconsin, Milwaukee

TIME FOR SELF-ASSESSMENT

Many students who have a hard time obtaining interviews to American M.D. schools ask whether it is better to attend a Caribbean medical school or an American osteopathic school. No question: Attend the American D.O. program if you are accepted to one. As I've described, with a few exceptions, your options as a physician will be essentially the same, graduating from either an allopathic or osteopathic medical school—and the two programs are growing even more similar.

But if you try your best applying to many American schools of both types and still strike out, consider why you are not getting accepted. If it is a chronic issue of your entire high school and college career resulting in a GPA much less than 3.5, or you really hate standardized, multiple-choice tests and got a low score on the MCAT, perhaps medical school is not the right choice for you. Trust me, it's not going to get any better. Medical school requires massive amounts of memorization and literally hundreds of multiple-choice exams, including the all-important USMLE board exams.

On the other hand, if your academic numbers are in line with those of matriculating American medical students and you still didn't get any medical school acceptance letters, consider how far you are getting in the process. If you are not even getting interviews, the rest of your application may be lacking. You may not have sufficient extracurricular experience; you may not be effectively describing why you want to go to medical school or that you know what you're getting into. These are very important to admissions officers. And with several applicants per available position, they can afford to be very picky.

If you *are* getting multiple interviews but still have not been accepted, then it might be your interviewing skills. Most undergraduate pre-med societies offer interviewing workshops. Try talking to someone who is in medical school or is a resident or practicing physician. Do some mock interviews and see if you can improve your skills. Alternatively, there may be some reason why medical school is not a good fit for you that is coming across in your interviews. An honest discussion with some practicing physicians may help you discover this.

Finally, it may just be bad luck and you need to try again. There are many applicants per position, so medical schools are often looking for specific blends of students, desiring certain percentages of nontraditional students, females, ethnic minorities, and the like. You may have just lost in the numbers game this year. If so, consider spending a year doing something interesting and hopefully related to medical research, practice, or education, then reapplying for the next year. It doesn't have to be research or volunteering at a hospital. Some people I know spent a year working as an emergency medical technician or a nursing assistant. Others interned at a medical device company or volunteered for medical mission work.

If at first you don't succeed in the process of getting accepted to medical school, you need to be honest with yourself about your weaknesses. Determine whether you are likely to have academic difficulties even if accepted or there are just a few things on your application that need improvement. Generally speaking, you should have no qualms about attending either an allopathic or osteopathic program. But think long and hard about attending a Caribbean school, given the high attrition rate and greater difficulty matching into a desired residency program. Many careers can be just as fulfilling and satisfying as being a physician, both in the health care field and beyond.

4.
ACCEPTED

"It Costs *How* Much to Become a Doctor?"

Congratulations! You've been accepted to medical school, and you're going to someday, hopefully, be a fully trained and employed physician. Now you have to figure out how to pay for it.

According to the AAMC, the median four-year cost of medical school (including expenses and books) in 2016 was $306,171 for private schools and $232,838 for public schools. Those numbers are up slightly since and will undoubtedly continue to rise.

If you're lucky, you have financially successful parents (or grandparents) who will pay for all or some of your medical education—or at least offer you an interest-free loan that can be repaid after you are done with training. Better yet, maybe you just inherited some trust fund that will pay for all of your med school plus expenses and still cover some kick-ass vacations. Though uncommon, there are scholarship opportunities, particularly for students with stellar academic performance, strong research interests, or underrepresented cultural backgrounds (essentially any ethnicity except Caucasian, East Asian, and Asian Indian).

STUDENT LOANS

For the rest of us, the friendly folks at the United States Department of Education will gladly lend hundreds of thousands of dollars to obtain a medical degree. These loans can be repaid over many years, at an interest rate set by Congress that changes every few years—as of this writing, 5.84 percent.

Unfortunately, since 2007 the federal government has become increasingly stingy with loans intended for graduate students, including med school loans. So-called subsidized loans that don't accumulate interest during school are now offered only to undergraduate students. And it's nearly impossible to fully get rid of student loans through declaring bankruptcy, even if you don't actually finish med school and residency—or if you suffer some sort of disability prior to being able to pay them off. This in part is why I caution against matriculating at a Caribbean medical school unless you are absolutely confident you will be able to finish and someday practice medicine in the United States. This is also why good disability insurance is critical as part of your overall financial planning.

If you're financially savvy at all, you've noticed that (again, as of this writing) you can get car loans for around 2 percent, but for some reason the federal government is charging 6 percent. This adds up quickly when your principal is over a quarter-million dollars. Private student loans do exist, but typically they are not a better deal except for post-training reconsolidation, which I'll talk about later. And one bit of protection you get with a government-issued loan is that, in the unlikely event of your death, the loan goes away and is not inherited by your next of kin.

Furthermore, the government loan servicers do offer a variety of options that can make the repayment process less painful, particularly during residency and fellowship. Income-based repayment (IBR) or Pay As You Earn (PAYE) repayment plans tie your expected monthly loan repayments to between 10 and 15 percent of your discretionary income. This is a reasonable amount to pay back during post-graduate training and can help minimize the amount of accrued interest during this period.

If you would prefer to just pretend your government-issued med school loans don't exist during residency, forbearance is still an option.

This allows you to avoid making any loan payments during your post-graduate medical training (that is, residency and fellowship)—but be aware that interest will continue to accrue the entire time. This can easily add $50,000 or more to your total loan amount by the time you're done with training.

Unfortunately, in yet another strike against physicians, in 2009 the government did away with deferment options for medical school loans. This option previously allowed nonpayment of loans during medical training *with* the added bonus of no accrual of interest. Nowadays it's probably a better financial strategy to go with the income-based repayment or just go into forbearance during post-graduate training and try to chip away as much as you can. There is no penalty for early repayment, so you can always choose the lowest monthly repayment amount (including nothing in the case of forbearance) and pay whatever you feel comfortable with each month.

Finally, there are some options available to forgive remaining medical school loans after a period of time working in underserved areas or in the public sector, such as an academic institution. The Public Service Loan Forgiveness (PSLF) program offers this, but this program's future has been a bit up in the air in recent years, and I'm not sure where it will stand by the time this book gets to print. In short, this program requires you to use the income-based repayment option on your student loans for at least ten years while you work in an underserved area at a public institution (such as a county hospital or academic center), at which point you may be able to write off most or all of your remaining loans.

Once you are an attending physician and making the big bucks, there are some relatively new options for reconsolidating your loans at lower interest rates, assuming your credit history is good. A quick internet search on "medical school loan reconsolidation" will produce relevant results. Most of these private companies are geared toward highly paid professionals with large amounts of student debt but otherwise good credit histories. They tend to offer more reasonable rates, somewhat flexible repayment structures, and no penalty for paying off early. However, if you have a family, you will likely want to obtain additional life insurance or some other protection, as should you die prematurely you will lose the forgiveness protection associated with the government-issued loans.

Okay, so what if you want to entirely avoid the painful process of taking out loans equivalent to a home mortgage to finance your medical education? Are there any other options?

I've already mentioned some of the obvious ones. You can ask your parents, close relatives, or some other benefactor. But you would probably already know if such an option were available to you. And you might be surprised to learn, as you go through medical school, how often this option is used! It is one of the few disparities among medical school graduates throughout their early careers—the rarely discussed difference between young practicing physicians *with* and *without* medical school debt. The perceived financial freedom and ability to choose specialty, practice location, and nontraditional training paths without considering massive amounts of debt after medical school can differ dramatically between these two groups.

If largesse isn't available to you, there are still a few other options that will be presented to you early in your medical school career, with varying degrees of sales pressure.

MD-PhD SCHOLARSHIPS:
MEDICAL SCIENTIST TRAINING PROGRAM

Most large medical schools offer a version of the Medical Scientist Training Program (MSTP). These are grants, supported by the federal government to encourage training of medical scientists, that typically pay for all of your education expenses in addition to a modest stipend for living expenses, travel, and supplies. In exchange, you agree to complete a medical degree and PhD in a relevant field. Acceptance into this program is competitive, and you are unlikely to be accepted unless you have a clear track record of research and an equally clear vision of why you want to spend roughly a decade of your life to obtain both degrees—and what you want to do with them. In short, don't even consider this option if your primary interest is to avoid student loans. It's not at all worth it unless you are truly committed to a career in medically oriented research. You will hate your life when you return to your med school rotations after finally finishing your PhD, only to discover that some of your new attending physicians (earning far more than your stipend) are your former classmates!

MILITARY SCHOLARSHIPS:
HEALTH PROFESSIONS SCHOLARSHIP PROGRAM

Newly accepted and first-year med students are routinely contacted by recruiters from all branches of the armed services. Such recruiters frequently host lunches and information sessions touting the benefits of the Health Professions Scholarship Program (HPSP), the most common way physicians get the U.S. military to pay for their medical educations. A recruiter will surely be willing to go over all the details with you. But in a nutshell, the deal goes something like this. You can sign up prior to starting med school or at any point during your medical education. Once you're in the program, your tuition is paid for entirely, and you will also receive a signing bonus, an officer's salary, and a generous allowance for books and supplies. While in training, you will be expected to attend a few military activities, including a modified boot camp and basic skills courses. Otherwise, most of your medical education goes uninterrupted.

The big payment comes *after* med school, and it often starts immediately upon starting residency. The general rule is that for each year of training paid for by the military, you owe one year of active service to the military. For example, if you were to join the HPSP upon matriculating in medical school, complete four years of medical school on the military's dime, then complete four years of residency (including your intern year), upon completion of residency you would owe four additional years of active duty service to the military.

One catch is that, depending on the specific branch of the military that you join, the odds of having your post-graduate training interrupted can vary. Historically, the Navy most commonly requires trainees to serve as a general medical officer (GMO) in a location of their choosing upon completion of their intern year—delaying completion of residency by the number of years required to serve as a GMO. Furthermore, for all branches, senior medical students must enter residency match for *both* military and civilian programs, and if they match in a military program, they must enroll in that program. Civilian programs can be selected only after receiving a deferment from the military match.

Finally, the old saying that "home is where the military sends you" is just as true in the HPSP as it is with traditional military personnel. Once done with residency, you will repay your years of service to the military wherever they choose. And that may or may not be in an active war zone, depending on the situation in the world and military needs. You may luck out and end up in San Diego for four years, or you may end up in the front lines somewhere—or in some town you've never heard of in Flyover Country. If you're young and unattached and looking for adventure, this may sound like an awesome opportunity. But if you have a family, a spouse with a job, or other roots that are deeper in the ground, this may sound like a huge headache.

However, from talking to several people who went through the HPSP, my impression is that it's rare to be barred from pursuing the specialty of your choice. I've never heard of it happening nor met anybody to whom it happened. And the one recruiter I actually met with prior to starting medical school assured me this hardly ever occurred. But nobody could ever quite tell me it *never* happens. After all, signing on the dotted line with the military is quite different from getting a job at Walmart. They pretty much own you until your payback is complete, and you never know what's going to happen out there.

In summary, my overall impression of using the military's HPSP to avoid incurring massive amounts of student debt for med school is that it is an excellent option for students who are already interested in serving in the military, especially those interested in a long-term career with the military including retirement as an officer. Though this certainly may change, the military currently offers very generous pension programs whose benefits increase with the number of years in service. While being paid as an officer in medical school and residency, your years of service accumulate, adding to potential retirement benefits. However, I think the HPSP is a horrible idea for individuals who would never in a million years consider joining the military if not for the scholarship money.

Financially, the HPSP will most definitely make your life easier during med school and residency. You will have no interest accumulating on student loans, you will get a nice stipend during school and a decent salary during residency, and all of your books and equipment are paid for by Uncle Sam. However, you will likely make less money as a practicing physician in the military than you would in a more lucrative private setting, especially in higher-paid specialties with longer training programs that translate into longer active-duty repayment obligations.

Ultimately, it all depends on how much the financial relief is worth to you when weighed against the loss of freedom and potential risk of being deployed to a war zone. For those intrigued by military life and considering a military career, this may be a great trade-off. For others, the risk may far outweigh any scholarship money the military can offer.

GEOGRAPHIC REPAYMENTS:
UNDERSERVED AREA SCHOLARSHIPS

Most other medical school repayment programs are less organized than the MD-PhD or military routes and are based upon the idea that you can sometimes get other organizations to pay off most or all of your loans if you agree to work for a specified amount of time in an area where not many people would otherwise want to work. Hence the name I assign to this category: *geographic repayments*. For those of you old enough to remember the reference, this is what the fictional Dr. Joel Fleischman did in the wilds of Alaska on the TV show *Northern Exposure*.

These repayment options are much more variable than the MSTP or HPSP programs and really should be examined on a case-by-case basis. They can be generally divided into government programs and private loan forgiveness opportunities.

The former group includes loan repayment scholarships offered by the Indian Health Service (IHS), the National Health Service Corps (NHSC), and many individual states that have large, rural, underserved populations. These typically involve a minimum service obligation ranging from two to four years and will pay off between $40,000 and $150,000 of student loan debt.

The latter group includes private practice or employment opportunities for new physicians in rural or otherwise less desirable practice locations. For example, I know several colleagues who finished primary care residencies in Minnesota and received job offers for clinics in small rural communities of northern Minnesota and the Dakotas, which always struggle to attract new recruits. Along with generous salaries and vacation packages, these jobs offered loan forgiveness in exchange for minimum service obligations.

Three important points about geography-based loan repayment plans: First, these are often restricted to *primary care* specialties, which includes family practice, outpatient internal medicine or pediatrics (*not* hospitalists), and sometimes OB/GYN. You're less likely to find an orthopedic surgery position in a rural area offering any substantial loan forgiveness.

Second, the term "less desirable geographic location" typically means *very* rural and remote parts of the country, such as nonurban parts of the Northern Plains, Mountain West, or Southeast United States. You're not going to find a rural loan forgiveness program in Aspen. It also frequently includes very specific hospitals in inner-city locales that have largely uninsured, impoverished patient populations.

Finally, the same general theme applies to these loan forgiveness programs as to the military and MD-PhD options. These options are great for someone who already is considering moving back to the small farming community where they grew up or who has a passion for serving underserved communities such as Native Americans or inner-city minorities. If you've always dreamed of finishing medical training and immediately moving back to a suburb and working at a community practice within a quick drive of your top-rated school district, you'll probably find these options miserable and not worth the money. For everyone between these two extremes, you will have to perform a cost-benefit analysis on your own.

As with everything in this process, be sure to find at least one or two physicians who have actually signed up for—and ideally completed—whatever programs you are considering. It's not that military recruiters or government agents are intentionally *lying* to you. But they are, after all, recruiters; their primary goal is always to attract good applicants to their programs, whether that involves working for the military, at Indian reservations, or in academic facilities. They are virtually never physicians who have actually gone through all of this, and their information is almost always limited to what they have been told by their trainers and supervisors.

PART II

MEDICAL SCHOOL

5.

STARTING MED SCHOOL

First Day of Summer Camp!

So this is what you've been waiting for—your first day of medical school! What's it going to be like? Will you head straight to the cadaver lab on day one? Will there be a pop quiz right away to separate the gunners from the questionable admits? (I'll talk about *gunners* later.) Will there be some sappy orientation with a crusty professor telling you that when he went to med school, only half of matriculating students graduated?

The answer is probably some combination of the above, but your first day will most assuredly *not* be stressful and will most likely have a nostalgic, "we're all in this together" tone—which probably isn't a bad thing. Starting medical school is stressful enough. A nail-biter exam or diving headfirst into a cadaver dissection really isn't necessary.

Details of your first day will vary, but in general, there is at least one day dominated by orientation activities. Since you likely interviewed at multiple schools and did so almost a year ago, you will get reacquainted with the lecture rooms, labs, lockers, and some of the deans and faculty. There will be lectures reassuring you that you are among the best and the brightest academically and that everyone in the medical school is there to help you succeed. And for the most part, this is true.

MED STUDENT DEMOGRAPHICS

One of the first things you'll notice about your new surroundings is that socially, medical school is much more like high school than like college, especially if you went to a large state college with tens of thousands of students on campus. You'll no longer have different people in every class, meet hundreds of new people each semester, and be regularly exposed to people from many walks of life with very different career paths and life goals.

According to the AAMC, in 2013 the average American medical school class had 134 students. A handful of schools are much smaller— such as Mayo, with around four dozen students per class—while others are much larger, such as a few state schools with class sizes in excess of 300 students. Most suburban high schools these days have class sizes much larger.

Also unlike a large, diverse college class, almost everyone you meet on your first day of medical school will have many things in common. Most obviously, all of you want to be physicians—and almost all of you will complete this goal. Everyone you meet will be very intelligent and very good students. Most will have been among the top of their classes all the way through school. A large percentage have known they want to be physicians for many years. And at most schools, at least 15 to 20 percent have at least one physician in their immediate family.

While the diversity of med school classes *has* increased compared to twenty years ago, many traits of matriculates remain stereotypical. It is certainly not a requirement these days to get a science degree in undergrad, and medical schools sometimes give preference to students with unique undergraduate backgrounds. But the vast majority of students still have an undergraduate degree in biology, chemistry, biochemistry, or some other life science.

The average age of a matriculating medical student is no longer twenty-two, but it still hovers in the mid-twenties. With increased competition for medical school spots, the demand persists for applicants to have *life experiences* beyond coming from a good high school and college with stellar grades and some volunteer experience. An increasing number of students now come to medical school having alternative careers for a few years prior to deciding to become a physician, myself included. (I studied business in college, cofounded a small technology start-up, then headed back to school to complete my med school prerequisites. Throw in some white-collar work at an insurance agency, serving at an Italian restaurant, and two summers operating carnival rides, and you've got a flavor of my "life experiences.")

Others have known for years they wanted to become physicians but took time between college and applying for medical school to explore alternative interests, such as travel, artistic endeavors, overseas work, or research. There is the occasional student well outside this age range who leaves a bona fide career to become a physician in the latter half of life. But this is still the exception and not the norm.

Another element of the average medical school class that persists, for better or worse, is that most of your classmates will be from families with professional backgrounds and above-average incomes. While the ethnic diversity of medical school classes has increased in the last decade, graduating classes are still overwhelmingly white, with many Asian-Americans and very few African-Americans, Hispanics, or Native Americans. Perhaps most telling is that according to the AAMC, in 2005 almost 60 percent of new medical students came from families whose incomes were in the top quintile of American households. By contrast, only around 10 percent of new students came from families whose incomes were in the bottom 40 percent.

I'll leave it to the medical school admissions committees and public policy wonks to debate the pros and cons of these demographics. But suffice it to say, compared to your first day of college, you will probably spend most of the time your first day of medical school meeting a lot of people who are a lot like yourself. That's not necessarily a bad thing. In fact, it is probably one of the few times in your life when you can enjoy working with colleagues who are all among the most intelligent, educated, and committed to their professions.

SOCIAL DYNAMICS

Due to the relatively small class sizes, cliques are unavoidable, and smaller social groups inevitably emerge. Sometimes these are based on specialty interests, such as the group of jocks who all shoot hoops in the gym after class and can't wait to become orthopedic surgeons. Other times it's based on interest in international work or volunteerism, enrollment in an MD-PhD program, or marital and family status. To be sure, friend groups evolve, grow, and shrink, and are not as mutually exclusive as some of the worst examples from high school. But groups of study partners and post-exam partyers definitely develop over time.

Also unlike on a large college campus, the first two years of medical school are typically structured such that everyone in the class is doing the exact same thing at all times. Given the high value of the lecturers' time and the specific nature of academic topics, it wouldn't make sense to break the class up into multiple groups and have lectures repeated throughout the week.

Going back to the title of this chapter, much like summer camp, you will find yourself in the first two years of medical school surrounded by the same people everywhere you go. You will all have anatomy lab together, drink together after exams, eat lunch together, sit through countless lectures together, and go to academic ceremonies and events together, and many of you will eventually sleep together. You will inevitably get to know many of your medical school colleagues better than you have ever known or will ever know anyone else you work with in your life.

In medical school, you will spend thousands of hours together with your colleagues in classrooms, study halls, and hospital wards focused on common goals and tasks. The focus and intensity required to achieve those goals will result in some of the most mentally and physically draining times of your life. It will challenge your preexisting friendships, relationships, and hobbies. But at the same time, it will produce some of the closest friendships and best memories you will ever acquire.

SIX DEGREES OF SEXUAL SEPARATION

With all the medical dramas like *Grey's Anatomy*, *ER*, and *Private Practice*, I am frequently asked whether the sex lives of medical students and residents are as fascinating as they seem on TV. As I said earlier in the book, it's unfortunately true that the comedy *Scrubs* is actually one of the most accurate depictions of life as a med student or resident on TV in recent decades. And as with most things on the show, I'd say it also provides a pretty accurate picture of the sex lives of medical trainees. I slept in call rooms in at least two dozen hospitals during my medical training, and I can't say I've ever witnessed an orgy of physicians and nurses stumbling out of a call room, everyone adjusting their scrubs with hair askew. So is it as steamy as some of the more dramatic medical shows make it out to be? Probably not. Are call rooms used for isolated conjugal visits? Of course. Are such encounters frequently interrupted by a code pager going off or a nurse calling about reduced urine output? Most definitely. Talk about killing the mood!

The most apt way I would describe sex among medical students is that among the single men and women—and for better or worse, some of the not-so-single men and women—everyone is connected by no more than six degrees of separation.

Medical school is an all-absorbing process very much akin to a small, secluded summer camp. Usually between one and two hundred students spend almost all their waking hours together—if not physically, at least in mind and spirit. They study the same materials, cram for the same exams, and stay up until midnight in the cadaver labs—reviewing anatomy, comparing residency plans, and talking about upcoming exams. Even the most social medical student will, at times in her training, become a complete bore to almost everyone else in her life, unable to form a complete sentence that isn't somehow related to medicine.

With so much time together and so many common points of discussion, it's inevitable that student romances occur—and they always do. But with such busy schedules and such strong egos and personalities, it's also inevitable that many of these student romances quickly fall apart—and they often do.

So by the end of the first two years of med school, I really do think you could have charted out a graph that would prove six or fewer degrees of sexual separation among all of my classmates who did not remain in committed relationships. Some of these relationships ended up in marriage, and many of my friends from med school whose weddings I attended are now having children and are getting along splendidly. Other relationships were perhaps just a nice study break and release from the isolation, pressure, and stress of med school.

As I said, just like summer camp.

6.
RELATIONSHIP ADVICE

Med School Years

After finishing the last chapter talking about med students' sex lives, I can't help but segue into a chapter about the hefty toll medical training often takes on preexisting relationships and marriages. If you're going into medical school with a significant other, you should pay special attention.

STATS AND FIGURES

The percentages vary from year to year and between schools, but my incoming med school class could likely have been split evenly into three groups. The first, slightly larger than the other two, included students who were purely single—or at most casually dating. The second consisted of students in serious relationships but not yet married or with children. The third included married students, with or without children. Of course, four years is a long time, and as med school progressed the percentages definitely shifted in favor of relationships, marriages, and children.

Data on this subject are hard to come by, but I've observed that med schools in large, expensive cities like New York, Chicago, or San Francisco tend to have slightly more incoming students who are single without children. Conversely, med schools in more suburban or rural settings tend to attract more families and married couples. But relationships inevitably blossom among med students—both with "outsiders" not in the medical profession and with fellow students. I entered med school having recently moved in with a serious girlfriend whom I had been dating for just over a year; I proposed toward the end of my first year, and we married during my final year. We experienced many of the challenges common to medical student relationships, so I'm not writing solely as a neutral observer.

Medical training and breakups go together like love and marriage, or so the stereotype suggests. And true to the stereotype, by the end of my time in med school I had witnessed many long-standing relationships broken, marriages ended in divorce, and engagements called off. One extreme example was a student who had been married for nearly two decades and got divorced after being accepted to residency out of state.

Though affairs may have been involved in some of these cases, I didn't get the impression that the cause was typically a clandestine relationship between attached students and their colleagues. More likely, medical school is simply a massive stressor of preexisting relationships that some couples survive and others don't. It is probably akin to the more common marital stressors of financial hardship, geographic moves, or problems in the bedroom. And sure enough, medical school often includes all three of these things!

A study published in the *Journal of Sexual Medicine* in 2008 examined the sex lives of students at a single medical school and found that 30 percent of men reported periods of erectile dysfunction, with 28 percent of men and women reporting significant dissatisfaction with their sex lives. According to the study, these numbers are all much higher than reported values from the overall population of men and women in their twenties.

MED SCHOOL STRESSORS

For couples that are married or in committed relationships before one or both of the partners starts medical school, many challenges immediately become apparent. Moving to a new city or state is often required, which can leave the nonstudent partner socially isolated, while the med student has an automatic friend source in his or her colleagues. Tuition bills and escalating student loans impose a tremendous financial burden. Finally, from day one of medical school, the student's time is aggressively taken away from the relationship by the requirements of studying, exams, lectures, labs, ward rotations, and eventually flying around the country interviewing at residencies. Meanwhile, all these days of intense studying and work are punctuated by post-exam parties and bar crawls occurring at odd hours and days of the week. If the non-student partner is employed in a more traditional job, the irregularity and randomness of the med student's schedule can be particularly disruptive. All of this can easily stress a young relationship.

Sometimes it's not just the obvious stressors that cause relationships to fail. The new responsibilities and challenges of medical school can also change one's identity and sense of self. Despite some pre-meds' hopes, medicine is hardly ever *just a job*; it is a career that can easily consume one's life and time, especially in the training years. Many couples will come into med school previously accustomed to both partners coming home at a normal time in the evening, having some dinner and drinks with conversation, then watching TV for a bit before heading to bed. The medical student's inability to leave work at the workplace and focus on the relationship and domestic issues when at home is often difficult for both partners to accept.

Finally, for couples previously accustomed to two incomes and normal working hours, the mere fact that one individual is now a student likely working more hours than in their previous position, making no money, and instead paying tens of thousands in tuition each year—and in the latter years of med school frequently having to work weekends, nights, and long days in the hospital—can be more than the relationship can handle. The nonmedical partner often feels this is more than he or she bargained for, and the medical partner often feels that the significant other's constant complaints and desire for more attention are more than he or she can handle on top of the already tremendous stress associated with obtaining a medical education. Each party becomes resentful of the other for different reasons.

WORDS OF ADVICE AND CAUTION

I want to assure those entering medical school in a committed relationship that you *can* emerge intact and still happily together. I saw many examples of surviving relationships among my medical classmates. But I also saw many relationships that didn't survive. Sometimes the breakup was obvious and expected by everyone. Other times, announcements of a severed engagement or impending divorce seemed to come out of nowhere.

My best advice is to talk to your partner well before you start medical school about how things may change in your lives and relationship once you start down that long and challenging path. Both parties need to realize it will be almost a decade before life approaches being "back to normal," and that it may never be quite the same. Nearly every physician is going to work more hours than the average American. And there will almost always be nights spent at the hospital, weekends on call, and evenings where dinner gets cold because a case goes long in the operating room or there are unexpected add-ons in clinic. Even after training, it's hardly ever a nine-to-five job, and that needs to be understood from day one.

For couples in which one is in medical school and the other is not, I recommend introducing the nonmedical partner to people in the same situation, either by seeking friendships with colleagues in similar relationships or by finding groups at your medical school for spouses and significant others. Not all medical schools have such groups, but I know my wife thoroughly enjoyed and appreciated the camaraderie and friendships made by the Resident Spouse Association where I did residency. Being a nonmedical person in a relationship with a medical trainee is a challenging position often best understood by others in the same boat.

If both partners are entering medical school, there will be additional challenges. First is the difficult task of getting both partners accepted to the same medical school—or at least two schools within close geographic proximity. Second, schedules will typically work out nicely in the first two years but can become impossible to coordinate once both students start ward rotations. While one person is on overnight call, the other might be home alone—and on and on, like ships passing in the night. Finally, there is the challenge of navigating the Couples Match in residency and then the vagaries of differing time schedules and geographic preferences when it comes to finding permanent jobs. Nevertheless, I know many couples in this situation who made it through all the ups and downs and are now happily married, both working as physicians and starting families. Where there's a will, there's a way. The shared understanding of being a physician can strengthen such dual-physician partnerships, but the many challenges will also expose any weaknesses.

For any parents, children always make things more interesting—and more complicated. Typically, the process of preparing for medical school is so time- and energy-consuming that most students in relationships delay having children until late in medical school or afterward in residency or fellowship when things are a bit more stable—though seldom easier. I did know a few classmates with children at home. In most cases, the nonmedical partner was the primary caretaker of the children. I knew of no situations in which both partners were in medical school with children, but it seems day care would likely be prohibitively expensive and difficult to coordinate with both parents having erratic and unpredictable schedules. Attending medical school and subsequent training in a city with helpful and available family nearby seems almost imperative.

ANOTHER DOC'S SHOES:
MED SCHOOL, MARRIAGE, AND MOTHERHOOD

By my first year of medical school I had been married for half a decade, already had a toddler in tow, and was two months pregnant with my second child. My classmates were on average eight years younger than me, scored three points higher than me on the MCATs, and overwhelmingly were single.

I wasn't alone in my journey. There were probably half a dozen of us "non-traditional" students in a class of about 180. We were for the most part older and with children. Many of us had left behind established careers and had spouses who suddenly became primary caregiver, housekeeper, and income earner. We easily identified fellow parents among our classmates. We were the ones with wrinkled clothes, bags under our eyes, and Cheerios in our hair. We toted pictures of our children—and carried guilt in our hearts for not being with them.

You will hear many examples of what we parents missed during medical school: ad hoc study groups, late-night fraternity parties (yes, these actually exist), skipping lectures to sleep in, and study-abroad mission trips. What you don't often hear is how we were class experts on childhood development, how we comfortably communicated with pediatric patients and their parents, and how our newborns prepared us for twenty-four-hour call shifts. Our single mates never experienced the merriment of a family happy dance after passing their first board exams. They never looked into the eyes of a mother in the final throes of labor and exchanged understanding without saying a word. They never came home crying after caring for a terminally ill five-year-old—to be themselves comforted by the embrace of small, yet powerful arms.

LIZ MEDINA ALM, M.D., M.P.H.
MEDICAL SCHOOL AND RESIDENCY: University of Minnesota, Minneapolis

Most of my classmates who had children typically were closest friends with other students in relationships with children. Recall my advice to find a spouse's group or other classmates with spouses or significant others not in the medical field; this is even truer for couples in which the nonmedical partner is predominantly at home with the children. Staying at home taking care of children while one's partner is spending long hours studying and at the hospital can be very socially isolating, and having friends in similar situations can make all the difference.

Make no mistake: starting medical school is not at all like going to a master's program for two years. Medical training is at minimum a seven-year journey, often occupying the trainee for eighty or more hours per week, with frequent work required overnight and on weekends. Furthermore, much of the student's time at home will be absorbed by independent study and preparation for countless exams. If your relationship has previously been in the context of both partners working normal hours in college or office jobs, it will be a dramatic change. You should be prepared for this and discuss how you will handle it ahead of time.

7.
STEREOTYPES AND SPECIALTIES

Jocks, Nine-to-Fivers, Geniuses, and Do-Gooders

Between my second and third years of medical school, when I was a teaching assistant (TA) for the first-year gross anatomy lab, I got to know the students in my lab room fairly well. I learned how they were finding the experience of medical school so far, why they wanted to become physicians, and their long-term plans. Much to my surprise, I could almost count on one hand the number of unique specialties the forty students in my lab intended to pursue. Nearly all were pining for orthopedic surgery, dermatology, neurosurgery, or family practice. Since I'm horrible with names, I employed my med student mnemonic magic and crudely divided my wide-eyed first-year lab students into four groups: jocks, nine-to-fivers, geniuses, and do-gooders.

DECISIONS, DECISIONS

As of 2016, the Accreditation Council for Graduate Medical Education (ACGME) recognized 165 specialties and subspecialties that newly minted physicians can specialize in. By the end of the third year or early in the fourth year of med school, most students have finalized an intended specialty choice. From there, it's up to each student's competitiveness and the luck of the residency match to determine whether they end up in their specialty of choice.

Students often take a complex and serpentine path in discovering their specialty. Most start with a general idea of whether they want to do something procedurally based or more cerebral in nature. Some know right away that they want to work with children or in the operating room. But over the first two years of classroom work and the final two years of experiential rotations through virtually all major specialties of medicine, many change their minds. Others find their talents are better suited for different specialties. And sometimes, unfortunately, students find they are not academically competitive enough for their intended specialties. Thankfully, most everyone eventually settles into a satisfying career.

What impressed me after talking to those first-year medical students was how little most of them knew about the myriad specialty choices available to them—and how just a few specialties seemed to dominate the list of intended fields of study. Granted, most twenty-something med students have had limited personal experiences in medicine, given their youth and usually good health. Still, even as an oh-so-wise third-year medical student, I felt the naiveté was excessive.

THE JOCKS

These students, mostly men, were destined to be orthopedic surgeons. This is perhaps the most blatant stereotype, but there is definitely some truth to it. Most med students spent the bulk of their time in high school in the library and not on the football field. But for the small percentage of incoming students who are reasonably athletic and love to talk sports, orthopedic surgery is a natural choice. The specialty offers the hands-on, fix-it opportunities of surgery combined with the ability to work with athletes—perhaps even as a professional sports team physician!

Of course, the vast majority of adult orthopedic surgery involves replacing knees and hips in our mostly sedentary and increasingly overweight, aging population. Furthermore, many of these orthopedic-bound students quickly realize that orthopedic surgery is one of the most competitive specialties around and requires top test scores, research, and excellent grades throughout medical school to match into the field. As such, some find they just can't get the numbers they need and choose another path. Still others discover they really don't care for the work or the surgical lifestyle.

There are many alternatives, and most of these orthopedic-bound jocks who don't match into orthopedic surgery find happiness in sports medicine, physical medicine and rehabilitation, or some other specialty that focuses on the medicine of movement. And while some of my closest medical friends are orthopedic surgeons, it's still amusing to recall the stereotypical behavior often displayed by ortho-bound folks: constant discussion of how awesome orthopedics is compared to all other specialties, bragging about shadowing experiences with team doctors, and scoffing at anything that doesn't involve bones or muscles. As much as you may want to rib them, remember that orthopedic surgery is a very competitive field, and many of these students are among the smartest in your class.

Finally, I want to make clear that while my description of the "stereotypical orthopedics resident" is indeed a stereotype—as are all the descriptions in this chapter—it is nonetheless grounded in reality. A 2015 report by the AAMC found that women make up 14 percent of orthopedic residents, despite a nearly fifty-fifty gender split among medical students. In my graduating class, only one of the nine students matching into orthopedics was female, consistent with that national average.

So what to do if you are interested in orthopedic surgery but don't fit the mold—you're not male, athletic, and sports-obsessed? Fear not! Residency program directors from specialties that tend to be dominated by a specific gender, ethnicity, or "type" of student most often line up with open arms to welcome a qualified applicant who breaks the stereotype. You should realize that in training and practice, you may frequently be the odd man (or woman) out. But so long as you are okay with this and get along with people in your chosen field, don't let it deter you.

NINE-TO-FIVERS

If one quarter of my anatomy lab wanted to go into orthopedic surgery, another quarter wanted to have all the perks of being a physician while enjoying a nine-to-five job after residency. These were the folks who imagined their post-residency lives being perfect blends of work, family, and personal time—the work happening in a sparkling, freshly scented clinic. These students wanted to become dermatologists, ophthalmologists, and otolaryngologists (ear, nose, and throat surgeons). I'm not joking; at least seven of my forty students said they were going into one of these three specialties. Not quite a quarter of the class, but still a completely disproportionate number. Only five students in my entire med school class of 209 people actually went into any of these three specialties.

Aside from being difficult to spell, the specialties focusing on the skin, the eyes, and the ears, nose, and throat have for many years been some of the most competitive specialties among American medical students. These are well-compensated specialties with manageable hours, not-so-onerous call, and hardly any emergencies—*and* there are very few residency spots in these fields. Most residency programs offer at most two or three residents per year in each of these fields. This produces a huge imbalance between the number of students wanting to enter these specialties and the number of residency spots available.

If you want to become a dermatologist, ophthalmologist, or otolaryngologist, you need to have near-perfect grades in all of your medical classes and rotations, achieve a top score on the USMLE, have some research in the field, and do away, "audition" rotations at institutions where you are considering applying. Obviously, the majority of students are not going to meet these criteria, and many quickly realize after the first few exams—and certainly after USMLE Step 1—that they are not going to be dermatologists, ophthalmologists, or otolaryngologists.

But fear not! Just as there are many alternatives to orthopedic surgery, there are several alternative specialties that are not as competitive but have similar attributes of a reasonable lifestyle with minimal overnight call duties and few emergencies. Examples include psychiatry, physical medicine and rehabilitation, radiology, and pathology. Some of these make up the so-called "ROAD" specialties: radiology, ophthalmology, anesthesiology, and dermatology—lumped together because of their supposed nine-to-five qualities. As an anesthesiologist myself, I would like to offer a more nuanced view of this. In addition to these "nine-to-five" specialties, there is a second class of specialties, unique among medicine in that they are *hospital-based*. Hospital-based specialties include anesthesiology, radiology, pathology, emergency medicine, and hospitalism. When these physicians leave the hospital, they can turn off their pagers and any thoughts about the events of the day and their patients. They are not the primary physician for any patient, so when they are not at the hospital performing their duties, they are entirely off duty. This is certainly not the case for most physicians!

Most physicians don't choose their specialties solely because of lifestyle or work hours. But this obviously is a large factor. For example, many students who come into medical school intending to become dermatologists or ophthalmologists ultimately realize they have absolutely no interest in the field, cannot match into the field, or are so passionate about something else—maybe even something with a far worse work-life balance—that they cannot help but pursue that specialty. Most physicians are committed enough to their careers and educations that they will sacrifice some practical things like lifestyle and income in favor of doing something that actually stimulates them intellectually and satisfies their career goals.

GENIUSES

The students I stereotypically assign to the "genius" category are not always those who ace USMLE Step 1 and go on to the most competitive specialties—though some of them will. Rather, these are the people who really *enjoy* memorizing massive amounts of information and learning as much as possible about medicine—purely for the sake of learning. Compared to most physicians and physicians-in-training, these folks derive an even greater amount of their self-worth and identity from their heightened intelligence and academic excellence.

These "genius" students are often drawn to cerebral, challenging specialties. Surgical fields include neurosurgery, transplant surgery, and cardiothoracic surgery. Medical fields include the more esoteric specialties, such as endocrinology, infectious disease, or nephrology. Radiation oncology is also a favorite of geniuses, highlighted by the fact that nearly a quarter of medical students who match into the field also have PhDs! I can't really say if radiation oncology is a medical or surgical field, because like most mere mortal physicians, I really have no clue what radiation oncologists do for a living.

DO-GOODERS

All incoming med students have some degree of altruism, but these guys take it to a whole other level. Some of these people were among my closest friends in medical school, because they are often the friendliest and most interesting, experienced, and genuine people around. You will find these students working with underprivileged populations, traveling abroad with medical mission trips, and getting involved in public health endeavors. Many join the American Medical Student Association (AMSA), the younger, more liberal version of the American Medical Association (AMA).

Specialties of choice for this group include family practice, pediatrics, internal medicine, geriatrics, and infectious disease. Those with a penchant for procedures gravitate toward pediatric surgery, transplant surgery, and sometimes plastic surgery with the goal of repairing congenital defects and burns. Many will tack on a master of public health degree at some point in their careers.

FINDING YOUR WAY

Obviously, all of the preceding is a gross generalization and shouldn't be taken too seriously. These are just observations made by yours truly over several years in leadership and mentoring roles in med school and residency. Just as different careers tend to attract people with certain characteristics and personalities, so you will find with medical specialties. And once a physician commits to a specialty, groupthink inevitably occurs, further melding the personalities within each field.

Early in your med school career, you may find yourself naturally drawn to one of the stereotypical specialties—and that's okay! But do keep in mind that one of the major goals of medical school is to expose students to the vast array of medical and surgical specialties. There are dozens of fields you never knew existed. Nuclear medicine, hyperbaric medicine, and occupational medicine come to mind. As you progress through training, always keep an open mind, and do what will make you happy.

If you're a happy physician, you will be a better physician, and your patients will benefit. That should always be the most important goal. You will only make yourself—and possibly your patients and coworkers— miserable if you choose a specialty because your friends have chosen it, because others expect you to, or because it's competitive and a challenge for you to overcome. Impressing your fellow students by matching into the most competitive specialty doesn't matter once you're a practicing physician. To be honest, it doesn't even matter once you're a resident. The moment you and your fellow graduates become residents, every last person in every specialty is thinking the same thing: "I can't wait to be done with this fucking residency!"

(Pardon my French, but there truly is no other word in the English language that so accurately describes the horrid beast known as residency.)

8.
GROSS ANATOMY

Coffee and Formaldehyde

My medical school featured an intensive six-week course in anatomy that served as everyone's first experience as a medical student. This was due in large part to logistics, since the formaldehyde-preserved tissues dry out over time, leaving them the consistency of beef jerky. A shorter, concentrated course allows for more effective learning from the cadavers.

DAILY ROUTINE

Each morning started with lecture in a large auditorium at 8:00, after which we all went to the locker rooms, changed into lab clothes (a mix of scrubs and old T-shirts), and headed to our assigned cadaver tables, which we shared in groups of four. We spent three hours in the lab, dissecting the cadavers and identifying structures. Most afternoons were free, but students usually spent at least a few hours each evening studying. Exams were every two weeks, focusing on extremities, thoracic and abdominal structures, and finally head and neck. A multiple-choice test was followed by a practical exam, during which dozens of students quietly traversed from cadaver to cadaver, clipboards in hand, writing down the names of each structure identified on the body.

The compressed nature of our gross anatomy course provided an excellent bonding experience for students and a "baptism by fire" initiation to the rigors of medical school. We were assigned our three "body buddies" at each cadaver table by alphabetical order, most groups consisting of two male and two female students. Contrary to the old days when physicians were exclusively men, med school class gender balance has been about 50-50 for at least a few decades. Body buddies didn't always end up being the best of friends, but the relationships were definitely intense. We spent at least twenty hours per week standing no more than a few feet from the same three people. We got to know each other pretty well—warts and all.

On a larger scale, the entire class bonded a great deal during those first six weeks. Attendance was required during morning anatomy lab sessions. And while several anatomy texts were available for at-home study, including the ubiquitous *Netter* diagrams, most students found it difficult to prepare for the practical exams without spending extra time with the cadavers each afternoon.

Many first-year students (myself included) came into med school accustomed to skating through high school and college classes with ease. Gross anatomy was the first time some of us had ever struggled or had to actively study for an exam. The information was thrown our way fast and furious. For some, the first exam served as a rude wake-up call. After that, even the students who had never sipped a beer their entire college careers came out to the bar to imbibe in a drink or two—or more.

FUTURE OF CADAVER LABS

The future of gross anatomy as a fundamental and core component of medical school is increasingly under debate. Many schools have already replaced the real cadaver-based anatomy course with virtual alternatives that rely on software and anatomic models to teach medical students anatomic structures and relationships. Others who haven't already made them are considering such changes.

There are several reasons, not the least of which is the tremendous cost of maintaining a cadaver program and laboratory. It requires massive resources to solicit and process donations, as well as a team of mortuary science faculty and students to preserve and maintain the cadavers. The sometimes laborious process of performing dissections also eats up a significant amount of time from the medical school curriculum, which is already under fire for its exploding cost to medical graduates.

Ethical concerns are also at play. The use of human cadavers in any form, including instruction of future doctors, dentists, and nurses, is under increasing scrutiny from human rights and ethics groups. Some argue the bodies are destroyed and desecrated in the process of dissection. Others say that given the widespread availability of computer-generated anatomic simulation models, there are far better uses for human bodies donated to medical research and science.

CADAVERS TEACH MORE THAN JUST ANATOMY

I don't know what the future holds for the decades-old institution of medical students first studying gross anatomy through cadaver dissection. All I can say is that at my medical school, most if not all students greatly appreciated the generous donations of their cadavers from the families of the deceased. Before even opening our cadaver workstation, each group of students was presented with a personal note written by the family of the deceased. These notes provided a story of the person's life, ways in which the medical field had touched them, and their motivations for wanting to donate their body for this purpose. We all attended a memorial service at the end of our gross anatomy course, at which various students presented donors' families with poems, letters, and other performances thanking them for their extraordinarily generous gifts.

The benefits of a traditional gross anatomy course became even more apparent to me at the start of my third year of medical school, when I served as an anatomy teaching assistant (TA). My own understanding of anatomy grew tremendously after spending countless hours in the lab each day with my fellow TAs, painstakingly creating "expert" prosections for students to review the next day. I witnessed firsthand the many intangible benefits working with cadavers provided to first-year medical students.

The process of becoming a physician is filled with experiences that challenge our perceptions and understanding of life and death. Most of the fresh-faced students who entered the cadaver lab on their first day of medical school had never been intimately involved with death. Even if they had been alive for the death of a loved one or friend, very few had ever seen a deceased body up close—and certainly most had never touched one and peered inside at the inner workings.

By the end of the first day of gross anatomy, students had spent roughly three hours carefully examining their cadavers, identifying external and internal structures, and moving arms and legs to see how various muscles interacted with bones, tendons, and ligaments to produce movement. By the end of the course, students had spent hundreds of hours with their cadavers, examining internal organs, nerves, fat, vasculature, and even the brain. This educational process was always approached with reverence and respect, and it was obvious to me how the experience transformed students' comfort in working with the human body and their understanding and appreciation of death.

And no, contrary to common perception, the first days of gross anatomy aren't filled with med students fainting at the sight of their cadavers, excusing themselves to settle queasy stomachs, or dropping out of med school in droves because they realized they can't handle the sight of a dead body. Everyone I worked with handled the experience professionally and with an appropriate amount of nervous anticipation and reverence.

I can't speak from personal experience about the relative benefits of a virtual gross anatomy course based on computer simulations, videos, and artificial or plastinated organs, but I can speak to the many intangible benefits to working with cadavers that are not possible with virtual models. Applying to medical school is competitive, so I don't recommend you spurn an interview or acceptance from a program that does not use cadavers. But it's a shame that this traditional part of medical education is increasingly endangered.

9.
PRECLINICAL YEARS

Drinking from a Fire Hydrant

In the early days of medical school, faculty and senior medical students often make the analogy that the first two years of med school (often called the "preclinical years") are "like drinking water from a fire hydrant." This is an accurate analogy for most folks. The sheer amount of information presented to students during the first two years of med school is unlike anything I ever experienced in undergraduate training. If a typical college semester consists of 15 credits, med school is like doubling down and taking 30 credits per semester. And with no fluff courses to lighten the load.

Most medical school curricula are divided into two distinct components: the preclinical and clinical years. The preclinical years are more like college, during which students can still amble into the lecture hall in jeans and T-shirts with a bell curve of tardiness. In fact, nowadays many schools video-record all lectures, making them available online for viewing from home. After the initial thrill of med school wanes, many students take advantage of this feature, and some of the dullest and earliest lectures have abysmal attendance levels. Personally, I found online viewing useful because I could speed up sections that I understood well (or that were taught by faculty who lectured so slowly they sounded like Ben Stein's teacher character in *Ferris Bueller's Day Off*) and repeat sections that were more difficult to understand.

THE DAILY ROUTINE

The typical med school schedule is Monday through Friday, with lectures running nonstop from 8:00 a.m. to noon with a few more hours in the afternoon. Later there are often labs, review sessions for upcoming exams, and optional information sessions (sometimes with free food to lure people in) about minimizing student loans, preparing for boards, or other relevant topics. Weekends were usually free, but I do remember a handful of Saturdays on which we had lectures or exams.

Not only do the lectures move along in rapid succession, but so do the exams. Each set of courses is typically just a few weeks long. There are sometimes midterms three or four weeks in. Other times the entire course grade depends upon one final exam. No more lounging around in lecture hall for a month or so before really buckling down for the exam. When one set of exams is done, you go out with your classmates to drink, commiserate, and generally blow off steam. And then you move on, because it's starting all over again. No rest for the weary.

NEW CHALLENGES AND EXPECTATIONS

I encountered some very bright students in my class who didn't seem at all fazed by the pace of the preclinical years. A gifted few still seemed to skate by with minimal studying—cramming a bit before each exam and acing everything with flying colors. But they were the exception, not the rule. Even if you are top of your class in high school and college and easily accepted to medical school, there is absolutely no guarantee that you will be anything but average among your new classmates—or even that you'll be average. I saw some very bright, hardworking students struggle to maintain average grades during med school. If you find yourself in this situation, get help as soon as possible. Every school has an educator or administrator whose primary job is to help students succeed in medical school.

Unfortunately, the rapid pace of the preclinical years is compounded by several distractions. Some are welcome—like forming new friendships and attending social activities, both organized and impromptu.

Others are not so welcome, including studying for the infamous USMLE Step 1—a.k.a. "the boards." Though the Step 1 exam is theoretically a comprehensive test of all the knowledge learned during the first two years of medical school, most students must review material and learn some new things that weren't well covered in the curriculum.

The big question of "What do I want to do when I grow up?" is a constant distraction for students during the first two years. Specialty choice isn't finalized until the fall of senior year, but most students start thinking about this far in advance. It is helpful to tailor early elective rotations to try out different specialties of interest. And if you seek a competitive specialty, early research and publications improve chances of a successful match.

Finally, as with most of medical school and residency, there are always annoying administrative details that bog students down. The process of applying for a medical license is worse than getting a home loan. Some schools require a DEA license, which can be equally annoying and expensive. And there are constant occupational safety requirements, including flu shots, respirator mask fittings, and PPD tests for tuberculosis exposure.

None of these things is horrible individually. But when piled on top of an already atrociously busy schedule, in which there never seems to be enough time to study all the required material, it's easy to understand why there are enterprising individuals who will do much of this paperwork for a price—and why some people (myself included, at my wife's urging) paid for such services during med school. You will find that in some cases, you *can* put a price on sanity.

Some advice you will appreciate later: a good habit is to scan into digital form every license, degree, immunization and health record, malpractice insurance document, and professional certificate you receive throughout medical school, residency, and fellowship. Start with your undergraduate degree. You will need to produce these documents many times throughout your medical career, when applying for training programs and jobs, credentials at hospitals, and state medical licenses. You will *not* enjoy having to dig through old records to find these things at the last minute.

NEVER ENOUGH TIME

I remember in middle school, high school, and even the majority of college, it was easy to assess all the material that could be tested on a given exam and estimate the amount of time required to study that material and sufficiently prepare for the test. For example, imagine a history midterm that covers American history during the Civil War and Reconstruction years. There are only so many dates, names, and places that can reasonably be tested. And depending on how quickly you can review notes and memorize material, you might set aside three hours of study time for two nights preceding the exam. You spend that time efficiently, and you can rest assured you'll do well on the exam.

For most people, the first two years of medical school completely blow that out of the water. At any given time you are always taking three to five courses, and that's done over a period of no more than a few weeks—maybe two months at most. Each day you have between four and eight hours of lectures, with additional material to read and memorize on your own. There is *always* more information that you could review, read, and memorize for an upcoming exam. And you could *always* use another few hours preparing for upcoming exams. Aside from the one weekend after each set of exams, there really are no times during the first two years of medical school when you can sit around and smugly feel that you are fully prepared for everything you are supposed to know at that moment. You will come to relish every last minute of those post-exam weekends.

THE VIRTUAL CLASSROOM

One might ask: if most schools record lectures and offer them online, why can't the same lectures be made available year after year—with the exception of updates for new or changed material? And if the first two years of medical school could be transformed to a mostly online curriculum, why does medical school have to be so expensive? Well, in the words of an old Baptist preacher, "Don't ask them types of questions, boy!" In all seriousness, most of the first two years of medical school probably *could* be boiled down to a few thousand hours of online lectures, with students coming to class periodically for proctored exams and attending afternoon labs and small-group sessions. From this perspective, the cost could surely be reduced.

But like most things in American medicine, you're not really paying for lectures, labs, or any itemized products when you pay medical school tuition. Deans of large medical schools are akin to corporate CEOs. The complex web of education, research, clinical work, patient care, and administration is far beyond the scope of this book, but suffice it to say that for the foreseeable future I don't see any positive news when it comes to reducing medical school tuition. And even if medical schools do start making better use of technology to reduce some of the recurring, tangible costs of medical education, you can rest assured that the savings will *not* be passed on to students.

OUTSIDE THE CLASSROOM

I don't mean to leave you with the impression that your first two years of medical school are filled with absolutely nothing but lectures and exams. To be more precise, your first two years of medical school are *mostly* filled with lectures and exams. Ninety-five percent may be an accurate figure. But med schools over the last decade or so have been gradually sneaking in more introductions to clinical life in the preclinical years.

Typically they set aside a few hours each month for group sessions that focus on the practical skills of performing a physical exam, interviewing patients, taking a complete medical history, and eventually performing less easily practiced techniques such as the breast exam, pelvic exam, and prostate exam. These "private parts" exams are usually taught with the help of so-called standardized patients who show up to willingly allow dozens of med students to approach them with shaky hands and a speculum. Most med schools pay these patients a small stipend, though it is sometimes a volunteer position. My experience is that most of these folks had some motivation other than money or altruism to volunteer for such work. For instance, many of the women had histories of breast or ovarian cancer, and nearly all the men had been diagnosed with or had family histories of prostate cancer. Don't worry: I've never heard of medical schools in recent decades that make students practice these exams on each other.

BEWARE THE GUNNER

Before I close this chapter on the preclinical years, I have one final definition for you if you don't already know the term. In your preclinical years you will first encounter the med school species known as a *gunner*—a student who starts his first day of medical school with both guns blazing, sporting a take-no-prisoners approach and attempting to outperform all of his peers whenever possible. It is precisely this type of student that led many American medical schools to adopt pass-fail grading policies and make class ranks difficult if not impossible to obtain.

There are obvious gunners—usually in the front row, raising their hands with gusto, highlighting their perfect dissections in anatomy lab, casually dropping hints about their recent publication in *Science*, and otherwise being obnoxious about how they're smarter than everyone else and are going to be the best physician in some ultracompetitive specialty, which is of course better than every other specialty. Thankfully, in my personal experience these folks were rare. My medical class was overwhelmingly cooperative and collegial. But there were some exceptions.

Even more dangerous are the *silent gunners*. These are the sleeper cells who live and work among you, unbeknownst to most of the class. When everyone else is out drinking at the nearest watering hole after a tough set of exams, these guys are already back in their apartments reviewing Step 1 keywords and pre-reading for the next set of classes. These guys are sneaking back into the anatomy lab before lecture to get in some extra studying. They're dangerous—and they might be sitting right next to you in lecture—if they even attend lecture.

10.
LAST SUMMER OF YOUR LIFE

Research, Missions, Travel, or Booze?

The preclinical years of medical school are more like college than anything else in the medical training process. Dress code is nonexistent. Attendance is for the most part optional. It's up to each student to prepare for exams however seems most effective. And there's a lot of day-drinking and celebration at odd hours following the end of each set of exams.

Another way the preclinical years are a lot like college is that there is actually a *summer*.

Most American medical schools give medical students two or three months during the summer between their first and second years of school to do whatever they please. This is absolutely the *last* time this opportunity ever exists, and what to do with that time has been a topic of angst for generations of neurotic, Type A medical students.

The main activity categories most med students partake in during the last summer of their lives are *research*, *missions*, *travel*, and *booze*.

RESEARCH

Research is typically the cheapest (it might even offer a paycheck!) and most "responsible" choice. This is what all the *really* smart med students do with their summers. (I chose this option.) These are the folks who win the lottery and immediately put all their winnings into savings accounts.

ANOTHER DOC'S SHOES: SUMMER AT THE OLIVE GARDEN

After that first year of med school, a very magical thing happens once the days get longer and the temperature rises: you experience "the last summer of your life"! Future doctors endlessly ponder what to do with the last three unstructured months of their lives, many choosing very practical things like shadowing a physician or volunteering abroad. I had a dream all throughout college that I had never quite found time to fulfill. At last I had my chance! I mentally prepared myself, did my research, and found the perfect job not far from home. The interview process was a blur, though I do recall possibly embellishing my level of experience in this particular trade. The next thing I knew, I got a phone call informing me I had the job. I was a bona fide Olive Garden waitress—and couldn't be happier!

Joking aside, I had always wanted to be a waitress or a bartender. It seemed like a rite of passage every member of society needed to go through. I figured I would get all the medical experience I needed over the next seven years (and I certainly did!), so I decided to spend this summer doing something completely unrelated to medicine. I was not the best waitress, and in fact was forbidden from working behind the bar once my manager realized I had absolutely no bartending experience. But I gained excellent life experience and met some wonderful people. If I had to go back and make the decision again, I would do so in a heartbeat. Waiting tables may not be what *you* choose to do with the "last summer of your life," but I encourage you to consider all your options and really take advantage of this golden nugget of a summer. Travel, spend time with family, do research, volunteer, run a marathon—do whatever makes you happy!

JENNIFER KICKENDAHL, M.D.
MEDICAL SCHOOL: Texas A&M College of Medicine, Bryan
RESIDENCY: Medical College of Wisconsin, Milwaukee

You may have absolutely no interest in doing research at any time in your professional career once you are done with medical training. However, many of the people who will be deciding whether you are a good candidate for their residency or fellowship programs do participate in research, and they like applicants who also participate in research. So keep your options open when it comes to future applications for residency and fellowship programs; it might not be a bad idea to get some research projects—and hopefully publications—on your curriculum vitae (CV—academic speak for "resume"—more about this in chapter 18).

That's the cynical, pragmatic view. But I actually have many positive things to say about choosing this option. And if you have research experience prior to medical school or are interested in pursuing a career in medical research, this option may be a no-brainer for you. Then again, if you already have some research experience but want to try something different, that's fine, too. In any event, I believe that all physicians, by the time they are finished with training—even if they are heading out to the middle of nowhere to practice general medicine at a tiny clinic—should have participated in medical research in some meaningful way.

This doesn't mean everyone needs to be first author on a randomized controlled trial or publish in a premier journal. But there is value in spending at least a couple of months working with a medical research team on one or more projects. That can mean participating in data collection or analysis, helping to write an actual paper, presenting a poster, or conducting bench research or animal studies in the lab.

If you're lucky, you can get a scholarship or stipend to help pay the bills during your summer of research. And if you're even luckier, your work will translate into a poster presentation or, even better, a legitimate publication that will forever be on your CV and a good talking point for residency and fellowship interviews. As I said, most residency and fellowship directors are academic physicians, and they love to see at least an interest in medical research.

If you're like I was at the time, with no prior research experience, don't fret. Many medical schools are research institutions and are filled with medical faculty just drooling for low-wage, hardworking medical students to do some grunt work for their research team. There are often websites or email lists at medical schools to facilitate such connections. If not, ask faculty about available positions.

Most summer research jobs are flexible and require ten to forty hours per week. These details can be arranged up front. At the time, it can seem like you're not accomplishing much, only entering data into spreadsheets or interviewing patients about pain scores. But over time, you will gain perspective on how medical research is actually conducted and what goes into the headlines you will read about for the rest of your career regarding some new drug, diet, or cancer risk.

Months or even years later, you may find out that your hard work has paid off and your project is being published in a journal, with your name among the authors! Even better, you may be offered the opportunity later in your med school career to write up the results of your project and become first author of a publication. You may even be surprised to discover you really like participating in medical research and want to incorporate it in your future career plans. At the very least, you will become a more critical reviewer of medical and scientific journals, which your patients will inevitably ask you about at some point.

MEDICAL MISSIONS

If the folks who put all their lottery winnings into savings choose to participate in research during the last summer of their lives, the folks who give all their lottery winnings to charity are the ones who choose to partake in medical missions.

Medical missions are organized trips by medical providers to third-world countries, typically lasting up to a few weeks. Teams consist of physicians, dentists, nurses, and some trainees including medical students. Participants usually pay their own way and also pay for supplies, but there are often scholarships available to medical students interested in such work.

This was a very popular option among my medical class, with many of my friends and colleagues traveling to places in South America, Africa, and Asia and assisting in handling patients and performing medical procedures to the best of their abilities. Often, students came back with experiences that would be difficult to achieve as a first-year medical student in the United States, such as administering vaccines, assisting surgical procedures, and suturing simple wounds. And of course, the cultural experiences in faraway places with very different living conditions are memories that many of my colleagues still remember vividly and that greatly influenced their career paths.

Medical mission work does have its critics. Some argue that the good provided to impoverished communities by a transient team of medical providers from an industrialized country is outweighed by the stress on local resources that comes with the team's rapid arrival and departure, as well as the need to dramatically change the arrangements of existing clinics to fit first-world medical expectations. There are also stories of visiting surgeons performing procedures on patients who later have complications that local physicians don't know how to treat, as well as patients being started on medications that are unavailable from local pharmacies. Some also question the use of medical students to perform tasks and procedures on third-world patients that they would not be allowed to do in their own countries.

However, most medical mission groups are well established, have good connections with local medical staff, and do as much as they can to minimize the negative effects while maximizing the amount of sustainable care provided to the local population. And virtually everyone I know who participated in this during medical school had positive things to say.

I do advise you not to plan this on your own. It's a complicated undertaking, and it's imperative that you use the available resources at your medical school and speak to others who have previously worked with specific groups you are interested in. If you attend a smaller medical school that doesn't have an international medicine facilitator, then search online for advice from other schools or practicing physicians. There is surely a faculty member at every medical school who has been involved with medical mission work at some point.

TRAVEL

Many students choose to spend the last summer of their lives going further into debt (or into their family's pocketbooks) with a final lengthy expedition to some exotic locale before the second year of medical school morphs into studying for USMLE Step 1, starting clinical rotations, applying for residency, and then losing three or more years of life in residency.

I'm sure you can conjure up a two- or three-week travel extravaganza just as easily as I can. Sometimes students travel solo with backpack in tow, exploring less frequently visited places like Vietnam, Uruguay, or India. Other students go with their significant others to resorts in the Caribbean or to romantic hotels in European capitals. For many young couples in medical school who have yet to procreate, this summer represents the last opportunity to travel without children and the massive time and financial constraints of residency.

The options are limited only by your imagination and finances. Travel certainly is a reasonable option, and it's one that can be spun into an educational, productive experience on residency applications and during interviews.

BOOZE

Finally, there's *booze*. This category doesn't actually have to involve massive amounts of drinking—though it sometimes does. Rather, this is a catchall that includes students who decide they are going to spend the last summer of their lives just enjoying themselves and relaxing. After all, it is the last big stretch of free time that most students will have until they are done with medical training—and quite possibly until retirement.

So how will you spend the last summer of your life: research, missions, travel, or booze? The decision is yours, but choose wisely! Once you start your second year of medical school, lack of free time will take on a whole new meaning that you've probably never experienced before. Trust me: at least once in the years to follow someone will try to make small talk by asking you what you do in your free time. And you will laugh.

11.
USMLE STEP 1

Choose Your Career!

Aside from the MCAT, perhaps no single exam is more important in defining the career path and opportunities of a physician than Step 1 of the USMLE, referred to by medical students everywhere simply as *Step 1*.

I've made many references to this exam already because it dictates so much of the early years of one's medical career, and its importance cannot be overstated. Once you have taken the MCAT and achieved a score suitable for entry into medical school, this is the only exam in the remainder of your medical career in which your grade can actually dictate your entire career path and specialty choice.

HISTORY LESSON

Back in the olden days, each American state had its own medical licensing exam that physicians had to pass before they could practice medicine in that state. This is similar to the way law board exams are administered by individual states, though the legal profession has also moved to a Multistate Bar Examination (MBE) now used by most states.

Obviously, this was a real pain in the butt, since a physician could graduate from medical school in Virginia and attend internship in the same state, requiring a Virginia license, then move to Louisiana for residency, requiring him or her to take another exam, then move to

Washington for fellowship, requiring yet another exam, and then establish practice in Rhode Island, requiring another exam.

States still require individual licenses, and make no mistake, obtaining state medical licenses is almost as onerous as taking individual licensing exams. But the process has been tremendously simplified with the creation of the USMLE; in most cases no additional exams are required for medical licensure in each state.

DETAILS AND LOGISTICS

The USMLE is actually a four-part exam, consisting of three computer-based, multiple-choice exams (Steps 1, 2 CK, and 3), as well as a simulated patient experience exam called Step 2 CS. Here we'll focus on Step 1.

USMLE Step 1 is a day-long multiple-choice exam that costs about $600 and is taken sometime toward the end of the second year of medical school at a commercial testing center. The USMLE website is very specific about which topics are covered:

- Anatomy
- Behavioral Sciences
- Biochemistry
- Microbiology
- Pathology
- Pharmacology
- Physiology
- Interdisciplinary Topics, such as Nutrition, Genetics, and Aging

The website provides an even more exhaustive list of specific material under each discipline that test-takers are expected to know. The exam content is certainly no secret, but the amount of information contained in that tidy syllabus is monumental. It literally includes almost everything taught in the first two years of medical school.

I won't belabor all the details of this exam, how to register for it, how to prepare for it, and how to take it. There are hundreds of books with hundreds—and in some cases thousands—of pages devoted to this topic. You can fly to some big city and take a thousand-dollar course devoted to this exam. Physicians have quit practice and made buckets of money telling other people how to ace this exam. That's not my goal.

But whether you are reading this book with just an inkling of interest in medical school or are already at some stage of medical education, it's not too early to understand the importance of this exam and the basics of how it works in the grand scheme of things.

MORE THAN JUST A LICENSING EXAM

USMLE Step 1 is intended to be a licensing exam—nothing more. It's not really supposed to be an evaluation of your performance in medical school or a deciding factor in residency admissions.

But it is both.

In fact, in many cases it is the *most important* factor in residency admissions. This isn't to say that if you score a really high score on USMLE Step 1, you're golden to go into whichever field of medicine you want and attend residency anywhere you choose. Rather, it's very often used as a cutoff criterion, such that a competitive residency program will specify a minimum USMLE Step 1 score that they want to consider for admissions review. If you scored below that number, your application will most likely never even be seen by an actual human being.

This situation stems from the fact that, as mentioned previously, medical schools over the last decade or so have largely done away with objective grades during the first two years of medical school, instead opting for pass-fail systems, sometimes with an "honors" grade to mark the highest performers. Medical schools have further obfuscated student performance by doing away with numerical class ranks and instead including vague adjectives in each student's dean's letter (a generic summary of each student's performance made available to residency directors for review).

With no grades and no class rank, how can a residency program director and admissions committee pick the best applicants in their pool?

Sure, there's research, extracurricular activities, scholarships, and awards. But what about sheer academic performance? No residency program wants to highly rank an applicant who may not pass their specialty board exam. And of course, every residency program wants to highly rank applicants who are among the best students in their medical classes.

The solution? USMLE Step 1. Currently it is the only objective way to rank and compare medical students by their mastery of content covered during the first two years of medical school—or at least the material the USMLE thinks should be covered.

Medical students everywhere—including many osteopathic students and international students wanting to practice in the United States—take this exam each year. Exams are batched together a few times a year, some sort of computer algorithm creates a grading curve based on each batch's results, and each test-taker gets a numerical score. As of 2017, a passing score for USMLE Step 1 was 192. It changes slightly each year, but it was 195 when I took the exam, so it appears to stay somewhere in the mid 190s.

I don't know what the minimum score is, but it's largely irrelevant, because if you fail Step 1, you've just narrowed your options so much it doesn't really matter if you got a 170 or a 180. The USMLE folks are similarly tight-lipped about a maximum score, but during my stint as a chief resident interviewing applicants to my residency program, the highest scores I saw tended to be in the 270s. Average scores vary each year, but the more important thing to look at is average scores per specialty by matched and unmatched applicants.

The folks at the National Residency Matching Program (NRMP) do a very nice job each year publishing data about applicants to all specialties, indicating the odds of successfully matching based on Step 1 scores, numbers of scientific publications, possession of other graduate degrees, and membership in the prestigious Alpha Omega Alpha honors society (which at many medical schools is partially based on Step 1 scores). You can take your application profile, plug in the numbers, and get a rough estimate of how many programs you need to apply to in order to have a certain chance of matching, based on numbers alone. Obviously, none of this guarantees anything.

But if you look at all these charts you'll see that you have far more options if you score very well on Step 1 than if you get an average score, a low passing score, or even worse, a failing score. You are limiting yourself to only a handful of specialties if you fail Step 1. I know people who even had immediate family members and scads of publications in competitive fields who failed Step 1 and couldn't get an interview.

NOT ALL SPECIALTIES ARE ALIKE

I've already identified a few competitive specialties, including orthopedic surgery, dermatology, and ophthalmology. What about the other specialties?

The easiest way to assess the competitiveness of medical specialties is by comparing average USMLE Step 1 scores of matched residents. These are the average scores of students who actually matched into each field. In general, the higher the score, the more competitive the specialty is. The table on the facing page presents the average scores for matching students from American medical schools in 2016, per the NRMP.

SPECIALTY	AVERAGE STEP 1 SCORE OF MATCHING U.S. STUDENTS
Plastic Surgery	250
Dermatology	249
Neurosurgery	249
Otolaryngology (Ear, Nose, and Throat Surgery)	248
Orthopedic Surgery	247
Radiation Oncology	247
Diagnostic Radiology	240
Vascular Surgery	239
Internal Medicine-Pediatrics (Combined Program)	236
General Surgery	235
Emergency Medicine	233
Internal Medicine	233
Pathology	233
Anesthesiology	232
Neurology	231
Pediatrics	230
Child Neurology	229
Obstetrics and Gynecology (OB/GYN)	229
Physical Medicine and Rehabilitation	226
Psychiatry	224
Family Medicine	224

Again according to the NRMP, in 2016 the average USMLE Step 1 score for all matching American medical students was 233. Clearly many specialties fall into this general range. More competitive specialties have average scores in the 240s, and less competitive specialties have average scores in the 200s. A handful of specialties that use a separate residency matching program are not included in the NRMP report—notably ophthalmology and urology, both of which are very competitive.

At this point, you might be thinking, "I just want to go into family medicine and practice in a small, community clinic somewhere. I don't want to go into a competitive specialty." That's fine, and you're entirely correct that you do not need to shoot for as high a Step 1 score as someone with his heart set on ENT or radiology. But know that Step 1 scores are still used even in less competitive specialties as cutoffs when reviewing applications, and a lower score will mean you can get into fewer residency programs than someone with a higher score. For example, you may have your heart set on an internal medicine residency at Massachusetts General, but if you scored only a 213 on Step 1, you'll probably be stuck at a lesser-known institution, potentially in a less desirable location.

PREPARE FOR SUCCESS THE FIRST TIME

If you want to do well on Step 1, start thinking about it during your first year of medical school. You can't wait until a few months before you take it to start preparing. Unless you are among the very brightest in your class, this strategy won't work. You may start out in med school convinced you want to do family practice (which doesn't require a stellar Step 1 score), but you never know where life will take you. By the middle of your second year, you may fall in love with the brain and decide your life will not be complete unless you are a neurosurgeon. All of a sudden you need to rock Step 1!

You might be thinking, "Isn't it just like the MCAT? If I'm not satisfied with my score the first time, can't I just take it again?"

Here's where the history and purpose of the exam make the situation unique. Remember, the USMLE is *not* intended to be used to evaluate applicants to residency—even though it is the *primary* tool used to compare and evaluate applicants to residency. It's intended to be used solely for licensing purposes. So the *only* way you can retake any portion of the USMLE is if you fail the exam—or if you passed it a long time ago and have to take it again for state licensing requirements.

In other words, you *cannot* retake Step 1 if you pass it but are not satisfied with your score. It doesn't matter if you had a bad day, fell asleep during the exam, or had to go to the bathroom too many times. You can, of course, cancel the exam at the testing center, citing some reason you couldn't complete it. In that scenario, it will cost you another $600 to take the exam again at a later date. But you can't complete an exam, get the score back, and then decide to take it again, as you can with the MCAT.

I hope I have impressed upon you the importance of this single exam—and of preparing early and doing well the first time you take it—since you can only take it once, unless you fail it the first time, which is never a good outcome.

How to do well on Step 1, pray tell?

That's a $64,000-dollar question, but the short answer is work hard. Apply yourself throughout all of your first two years of medical school as much as you possibly can. Do as well as you can on every exam you take, and try to follow along in each class with a Step 1 review book or the list of topics on the USMLE website. If specific topics are mentioned in the biochemistry section on the USMLE website, make sure you really understand those well when you're studying for your med school exams in that class. And if some topics mentioned on the USMLE topic list aren't covered in your med school class, feel free to ask your professor about them or at least study them on your own.

There are hundreds of Step 1 review books. Unless one of the publishers wants to pay me, I'm not going to endorse anyone here. You'll know within a few months of starting med school what the review book du jour is in your class. If not, ask the second-year students; they'll know. If it's popular, it's probably fine. But each does have its own style, so make sure you take a look before you purchase. Some are very terse, others more verbose. You might learn better from one style versus another. Think about what types of study materials have worked well for you in the past.

There are also audio courses, video courses, and real-life courses that require travel and major financial outlays. You may or may not find any of these things useful. If you took one of the MCAT review courses and loved it, you might want to consider a similar course for the USMLE. If you instead prefer holing up in your apartment and studying with a single book for a few months, that's your prerogative. Do whatever works for you, but keep at it and stay focused.

Finally, I cannot overstate the value of practicing with some sort of online or computer-based system that is similar if not identical to the actual test. Use the practice tests USMLE offers online to at least get a feel for how it works. Some private study courses boast interfaces very similar to the real thing. You don't need to use that as your primary study resource, but at least spend some time practicing taking questions on a computer in a timed setting, so the timing and structure of the exam are not a surprise to you when you get to the exam site.

The night before the exam, try to get some sleep and relax. I see no benefit at all in cramming for this exam. It's an all-day marathon, and the last thing you want to be is tired. The exam tests you on tens of thousands of pieces of information, covering virtually everything you learn in the first two years of medical school—a huge chunk of data. It takes months to adequately prepare for it. There is no way you are going to memorize or cram anything meaningful in one night to significantly improve your score.

AFTER THE EXAM

You've finished Step 1, had a few drinks to celebrate, taken a few more med school exams, and finally gotten your score back. Happy with your score? Congratulations! Go out and celebrate again! Not happy with your score? Uh-oh. Now what?

First, you need to assess the situation as objectively as possible. Have your friends and trusted advisers look at it too. If the average for people who match into your desired specialty is 240 and you got a 220 on your USMLE but are top of your class, with multiple first-author publications, that's one story. It's an entirely different story if you have marginally passed every single class in medical school, have minimal research experience, don't really have anything extraordinary on your CV (med school resume), and you got a 198.

Be honest with yourself and determine early on whether you can salvage the situation or should instead focus on finding a different, equally satisfying specialty. You might be surprised and discover as you progress further in your career that you actually like your second choice better than your first—or at least just as much. Think about what exactly drew you to your desired specialty in the first place and look for less competitive specialties with similar characteristics.

Were you interested in working with athletes but are way off the numbers to get into orthopedic surgery? Consider instead family medicine with a fellowship in sports medicine, or perhaps physical medicine and rehabilitation (PM&R). Did you have your heart set on dermatology for its predictable schedule and minimal emergencies? Consider psychiatry, PM&R, or pathology instead.

Being accepted to medical school doesn't guarantee your ability to practice your ideal medical specialty. However, most physicians leave residency satisfied with their choice of specialty.

If you instead decide to go into salvage mode to ensure your first choice of specialty, then you need to optimize every other piece of your application. Do as well as you possibly can in all your remaining preclinical work. Try to receive a grade of "honors" on as many of your clinical rotations as possible. Start preparing for Step 2 CK (more on that later), planning to take it early and ace it, so it will appear on your CV when you apply for the residency match. Get some research under your belt if you don't already have some on your CV. Do away ("audition") rotations in your desired specialty at programs you are interested in, and plan on performing solidly so you leave a good impression.

One more salvage maneuver is to try your best to be elected to the Alpha Omega Alpha (AOA) honors society (not to be confused with the American Osteopathic Association), one of medical school's oldest and most prestigious honors societies. Most schools elect two batches of students to be in the club, the first during their third year (called "Junior AOA" recipients) and the second during their fourth year (called "Senior AOA" recipients). Overall, "Junior AOA" is a bit *more* prestigious, because that means you already were up to snuff by the end of your second year. But both are excellent and will do wonders in helping you get into the residency of your choice. Residency directors *love* having a bunch of AOA students in their ranks.

INFORMATION FOR OSTEOPATHIC
AND INTERNATIONAL STUDENTS

Osteopathic medical students take a similar multistate licensing exam, called COMLEX-USA, administered by the National Board of Osteopathic Medical Examiners (NBOME). Sound familiar? It's basically the same thing as the USMLE, as per conversations from my osteopathic colleagues. But there is a twist! As I described in a previous chapter, the ACGME (Accreditation Council for Graduate Medical Education) and AOA (American Osteopathic Association) are in the process of merging their residency programs and application processes. The COMLEX-USA is unlikely to go away anytime soon, but the two licensing exams may eventually merge. In the meantime, know that osteopathic students applying to competitive residency programs have traditionally taken *both* the COMLEX-USA and the USMLE. This is so D.O. applicants can widen their net to include applications to ACGME residencies, which generally require the USMLE. So what I've said about the USMLE applies to osteopathic students, especially for competitive specialties.

If you are an international medical graduate (IMG), especially from a Caribbean school, the USMLE Step 1 exam is even more critical. You already have multiple strikes against you when applying to American residency programs as an IMG. Many residency directors have no idea how to assess a student from a foreign school, and they often view applicants from Caribbean schools with a jaundiced eye. It is *vital* that you level the playing field as much as possible by blowing Step 1 out of the water and scoring well above the average of American medical graduates accepted into your specialty of choice. With greater numbers of American medical school graduates over the last decade (with no concomitant increase in the number of residency spots), this is now critical even for traditionally less competitive specialties such as internal medicine, family medicine, and pediatrics.

12.

SHORT WHITE COAT

Now You're a *Real* Doctor (Almost)

Congratulations! You've survived the preclinical years and Step 1, and now you're donning your short white coat for the first time as you embark upon your first clinical rotation! Okay, maybe you put on the white coat for a ceremony and a few pretend doctor sessions in your first two years . . . but now it's for real! *Well . . . kind of . . .*

All joking aside, starting the third year of medical school truly is the beginning of an entirely different phase in your life as a medical student—and in your overall career as a physician. Most medical schools start clinical rotations during the summer of your second year, which becomes the beginning of your third year. See, I wasn't lying when I said the first summer of med school is the last summer of your life!

Gone are the days of showing up late to lectures in jeans and a grubby T-shirt, cramming for exam after exam, and meeting up after class with nearly your entire class to blow off steam at a bar. Now you're almost a *real* doctor! That means you need to start dressing up for work. You have to interact with real patients, other real doctors, nurses, a whole slew of technicians, and ancillary staff you never knew existed. You even have to start getting to work on time. And depending on the rotation, that can be really, really early! If you weren't a morning person before, you will be soon.

SCHEDULING CLINICAL ROTATIONS

There are two main approaches to scheduling clinical rotations for third- and fourth-year medical students. The process is typically completed at the end of the second year. Some med schools assign rotations in blocks, dividing the class into a few different groups, whose members follow a predefined core curriculum during the third year. This typically consists of the following basic disciplines:

- Internal Medicine
- General Surgery
- Pediatrics
- OB/GYN
- Neurology
- Psychiatry
- Primary Care

The other school of thought is to give students complete freedom in designing their schedule. This is usually facilitated by some sort of lottery system, in which various rounds of course selection take place, giving every student a fair shot to select their most desired courses at times and locations of their choosing.

Electives—such as radiology, emergency medicine, or urology—are sometimes allowed during the third year, even at schools that require a predefined curriculum, but this varies from place to place. In either system, the majority of electives are taken during the fourth year. But given the option, it's always a good idea to request electives in specialties that interest you as early as possible—even toward the end of the third year if allowed. This enables you to try out a specialty early in the process and decide if it's something you might want to pursue further as a possible career.

In fact, you should have two main goals during your clinical years. The first is to learn as much as you can about the basic clinical disciplines. This is the time to figure out how all the stuff you learned in the first two years actually applies to real medical practice, and to develop the foundation that will prepare you for residency. You will accomplish this goal by seeing patients, preparing for rounds and procedures, and studying for exams that will still haunt you every few weeks during your third year.

The second goal is to figure out what you want to do with your life. You should approach each rotation with as open a mind as possible. Consider each rotation a trial run of that specific field of study to see if it's something that interests you. Sure, you may know "for sure" that you want to be a family practice doc, but you never know! I witnessed many unexpected transformations in my medical class. People who knew they wanted to go into surgery ended up in internal medicine. Folks who were destined for radiology ended up doing OB/GYN. Sure, there were plenty who stuck to their guns. But you might be surprised by what you like when you try it.

FIRST DAY ON THE JOB

The first day of clinical rotations can be intimidating regardless of which rotation you are on. Students are especially intimidated by general surgery, OB/GYN, and other specialties to which they have had less exposure. Just remember, all of your superiors—interns, residents, fellows, and attending—were once in your shoes. Even the oldest faculty will have some memory of what it was like to be a tenderfoot, third-year medical student.

Speaking as someone who regularly worked with medical students as a resident and then a fellow, I can say that the best any of us hope for from a fresh third-year student is that you don't get in the way. If you can also occasionally help out by producing a stethoscope, pen, or recent lab value during rounds, then all the better.

Until you get your feet wet in a rotation and get a feel for the personalities involved, it's better to lay low and speak only when spoken to—or when you truly have something useful to add to the conversation. Don't try to be overly funny or amusing on your first few days.

And definitely don't try to show off or, even worse, show up your interns, residents, fellows, or attendings. At this stage of the game you really don't know anything—and nobody expects you to know anything. If you mouth off a bunch of garbage trying to act like you do know a lot, people will think you're an ass. And that's not a reputation you want to acquire early in the game.

The only exception is if someone is trying to remember some esoteric bacteria that came up in a culture report during rounds, and you distinctly remember the microbiology table from your recent studies for Step 1 that had all the bacteria listed by class and antimicrobial sensitivities. Sure, in that case, feel free to show off your Step 1 knowledge, because you will certainly know that better than anyone else in the room. Otherwise, a less-is-more approach is best.

PRETEND PLAY

Being a third-year med student on rotations is a lot like being a server-in-training at a restaurant. You know what I'm talking about: the awkward situation when you're seated in a restaurant and two servers approach, one behind the other. The one in back says nothing; the lead server introduces him or her as someone in training. Yeah, that's pretty much what it's like being a third-year med student. (Word of advice: If the attending physician fails to do so, it's always a good idea to introduce yourself to patients when observing clinical encounters. Nobody likes going to the doctor and wondering who the random person lurking in the background is.)

The purpose of clinical rotations is to pretend to be a doctor and learn from the experiences—in the same way a child plays pretend and learns how to be a real adult. Nobody really trusts much that a med student says about an interview or exam with a patient. Any critical finding will certainly be double-checked by a resident or attending. Even an unusual lab value reported by a student during rounds will likely be verified by someone more senior before any treatment decisions are made. For the third-year medical student, this is the last time you can make dumb mistakes, not really understand what's going on, and still get away with it.

Granted, you can't haphazardly make changes to an ICU patient's drips or unilaterally decide to cut a suture during surgery. Those types of actions would most likely land you in the dean's office, if not get you summarily dismissed. As I said, third-year medical students on rotations are to speak only when spoken to and to do only what they are told to do. Nothing more and nothing less.

Don't worry; you will gradually acquire some independent duties. You will "pre-round" at some godforsaken hour of the morning. That involves frantically going through the electronic medical record and collecting morning vitals and labs for all the patients. You might do an initial history and physical on new patients in the emergency room while your residents review the charts and put in initial orders. You might hold some retractors in the operating room and cut some sutures—usually too short or too long. You might even be given the coveted duty of writing a discharge summary. This is a task that will initially take you two hours and result in a novel that rivals *War and Peace*, compared to what will, by the end of your residency, be a five-line paragraph cranked out in six minutes.

The hours will sometimes be long, but the responsibilities are still minimal. You are mostly working with your resident team and occasionally interacting with your attending physicians (the real docs) to discuss patients, consider differential diagnoses, and formulate treatment plans. You will see firsthand how physicians think when narrowing down the massive list of possible diagnoses to a manageable few. You will witness how surgeons and anesthesiologists deal with unexpected disasters in the operating room. You will observe ER physicians managing chaos in the emergency room. And you will sit right next to an attending family practice physician while he explains to his lifelong patient that she has terminal cancer and has only a few months to live.

You will be the proverbial fly on the wall in virtually every possible realm of medicine, ranging from inpatient psychiatry wards and

OB/GYN delivery suites to outpatient clinics and radiology reading rooms. Though you sometimes may feel like you're not making an impact, this broad and intimate exposure to every single facet of medicine is what gives physicians a unique, universal perspective of the health care system and how all the pieces of medicine fit together in managing patients' health.

SHELF EXAMS AND PIMPING

Unfortunately, you're not yet out of the woods when it comes to taking frequent exams. It's not as bad as the preclinical years, during which you often sit for several exams each month. But it's still a constant burden. Each rotation typically lasts from two to eight weeks, depending on whether it is an elective or a core rotation. At the end of all core rotations and most electives, medical students are given some sort of exam. So-called shelf exams— standardized exams administered across the country—are frequently used for core rotations. The questions are very similar to those asked in the USMLE Step 2 and 3 exams, so they are good preparation. There is usually no designated study time during clinical rotations, so students must use some of their limited free time to prepare for these exams.

Students on clinical rotations are also frequently tested daily with so-called pimping from anybody above them on the academic medicine food chain—essentially everyone ranging from interns up to the attending physicians. Pimping in the medical field has nothing to do with prostitution; it is loosely based on the Socratic method of learning by inquiry. This can take the form of assigned readings the student is asked to summarize and present to the team the following morning; more typically, the student is asked an impromptu medical question, often in front of his or her peers during rounds or during a surgical procedure—say, about the possible causes of pancreatitis while the student is nervously tying a skin suture in the operating room. If the student answers correctly, a follow-up question of greater difficulty or depth will inevitably follow. This continues until the student doesn't know the answer. At this point, the resident or attending will ask related questions in attempt to lead the student to talk through his or her thought process, ultimately getting to the right answer. Eventually, something interrupts rounds or the surgeon needs to concentrate on the operation, and the pimping abruptly stops. The student either feels satisfied with his or her performance or wants to shrink to the size of a pea.

Now that I've been on the other side as a resident, fellow, and ultimately attending, I realize that half the time I don't even remember whether students or more junior residents get the answers right. It's really not all about getting the right answer, and half the time pimping attendings and residents don't really *expect* a student to get the right answer. It's all about the thought process involved in attempting to get to the answer and how well the student expresses this mental pathway.

I used to hate pimping, as do many medical students and residents. But over time (perhaps it was Stockholm syndrome), I came to accept the process as a standard form of interaction and eventually started using it with friends and loved ones—however, typically this was not appreciated, and I can't recommend it outside of the medical realm.

THINKING LIKE A DOCTOR

As you progress through the third year of medical school, you continue to learn the basic skills required to become a doctor. How do you present a patient in a succinct and understandable way, using precise medical terms and focusing on the most clinically relevant information? How do you explain diagnoses and treatment plans to patients? How do you formulate a manageable list of potential diagnoses (the so-called differential diagnosis) from a patient's history and physical exam findings? How do you come up with a treatment plan based on your differential diagnosis? How do you know when to consult medical colleagues or solicit the services of ancillary medical staff? How do you "code" a dying patient? How do you handle a septic patient in the ICU? When do you need to place invasive lines? How do you know when a patient is really sick and needs to be monitored more carefully?

How do you know when you can do nothing more to heal a patient and they are about to die?

None of these abilities come naturally to physicians. They are learned by observation, reading, studying, and interacting with patients, and by trial and error. It's a long process, and that's why it takes almost a decade to become a physician. Indeed, one of the last skills a physician masters is the ability to walk into a room and within seconds know if a patient is okay, critically ill, or actively dying.

As you reach the fourth year of medical school, you will start sub-internship rotations, or "sub-I's" for short. Sub-internships are so named because at this point, medical students are expected to be "almost interns." You will be expected to truly own your patients—though still with resident and attending oversight. You will take on sicker patients in critical care settings and emergency rooms. You will be the primary contact for the patient, examining the patient daily, keeping up on labs and vital signs, and presenting overnight events, active problems, and diagnoses and treatment plans for each patient during rounds. Your leash is a bit longer by now, and bad decisions or oversights can potentially cause bad outcomes.

But don't worry! So long as you always tell your interns, residents, or attendings above you anything you are concerned about, you are still generally off the hook. Everybody knows you still don't really know much about direct care, and you have several pairs of eyes double-checking your work all the way through the end of med school.

Throughout the preclinical years you are distracted by the specter of the USMLE Step 1 and figuring out what you want to do when you grow up; in the clinical years you are distracted by the looming complex and expensive process of actually applying to residency and ultimately learning where you are going to spend the next several years of your life. More about that later . . .

13.
DUAL-DEGREE PROGRAMS

Outlets for Overachievers

If you are attending a medical school with a combined MD-PhD program but are not in the program yourself, you may notice some colleagues you got to know well in the first two years of med school abruptly disappear somewhere around the start of clinical rotations. This is when most programs start the research years of the MD-PhD program, which takes three to six years, depending on how quickly one gets settled in a lab and starts a project, and then how smoothly the project goes and how expediently the student can prepare a PhD thesis. Only after completion of the PhD degree do students return to clinical rotations in med school.

During the PhD research years, you will occasionally see these students at school-wide events, at local eating establishments and watering holes, and walking the halls of adjacent lab buildings. But by and large, most of these folks will be out of sight and out of mind for several years, not to return to their clinical rotations until you are likely knee-deep in your intern year or even halfway through residency. In my case, I returned to my med school alma mater to do a fellowship after four years in a different state for residency. You can imagine my surprise when I ran into a few of my MD-PhD classmates who were still in their final years of med school while I was in my fifth post-graduate year of training. I am now an attending, completely done with training and board certified in both my specialty and subspecialty, and many of the

MD-PhD students I started out with are just in their first year or two of residency.

So I repeat: the integrated MD-PhD medical scientist program is *not* for the faint of heart. Nor is it for people with only a passing interest in research. And it *certainly* is not for people whose primary interest is getting the federal government to pay for their medical education. It is a long haul that adds several years to your time in medical school, and the potential income—not to mention years of your life—lost during those years is tremendous.

DUAL-DEGREE OPTIONS

So what if biomedical research isn't your bag, but you're still jonesing to tack on a second degree to the already illustrious medical degree? According to the Association of American Medical Colleges, you're not alone. Enrollment in dual-degree programs has increased 36 percent nationwide over the last decade. Just under 4,000 students pursued such programs in 2002, while over 5,300 did so in 2011. With a limited number of spots available, competition for these positions continues to increase.

One of the most popular dual-degree combinations is the MD-MPH, which bundles a master of public health degree with the M.D. This can be a useful addition for students interested in research or epidemiology, and of course incorporating a public health career in their practice. While one can apply to such programs prior to enrollment in med school, it isn't uncommon to apply to M.P.H. programs within the first few years of medical school. This option usually adds one year of training to the mix.

Far less common is the MD-JD combined degree, which adds a law degree to the M.D. This is a natural choice for students interested in becoming a malpractice attorney, but there are plenty of folks in that profession who do just fine without a medical degree. More realistically, this degree can help physicians segue into health care administration, public policy and government careers, or even jobs in forensic science.

This dual-degree program more commonly requires admission prior to enrollment, so plan ahead for this one. Most programs allow students to earn both degrees in six years, as opposed to the seven it would normally take someone to become both a lawyer and a physician.

An increasingly popular choice is the MD-MBA program. This adds a master of business administration degree to the M.D. in a total of five years versus the six years it would normally take to complete both programs. Many students come to medical school with little exposure to finance, marketing, and basic business concepts, so this degree can be a useful addition to physicians interested in eventually pursuing careers in health care administration, entrepreneurship, medical consulting, or academic leadership, or running a small private practice office. Most medical schools allow application to this program after admission, but given the increasing popularity of this program, planning ahead is advisable.

COSTS AND BENEFITS OF A SECOND DEGREE

Unlike the MD-PhD degree, which gives students scholarship money formally funded by the federal government, most of these other dual-degree programs are funded by their hosting universities. In many cases, students can get most or all of their second degree paid for—or at least included in the obscene amount already paid for the medical degree. This varies from school to school, however, so it's important to investigate this in advance.

Finally, it's important to keep things in perspective and honestly assess whether you will likely benefit from and use the knowledge and skills obtained from a second degree. A year or two of your life is no chump change when you're already committing nearly a decade to medical training. And while a second degree may help you land a traditional physician job in a very competitive field and a tight geographic market, in general this isn't necessary.

ANOTHER DOC'S SHOES: THE HEALING POWER OF CUTCO KNIVES

During college, I wanted to study business because I idealized the act of building a business, competing for success, and having freedom from arduous, fixed work hours. But I had doubts and wondered if my highest achievement would be selling a thousand more Cutco knives. I begrudgingly completed prerequisite coursework for med school—at the pleading of my parents, both physicians. In the end, I lacked the drive, money, and brilliant idea to start a business . . . so med school it was.

Part of me died the first year of med school. Fortunately, I am extremely good at memorizing things and did well academically, but I took no pleasure in regurgitating facts about organ systems, pharmacology, and "evidence-based" medical therapies. Some fire returned inside me when I learned of the joint MD-MBA program, which promised cool internship opportunities and courses in entrepreneurship, finance, and marketing. I was excited to see how the "other half" lived, sell a little snake oil, and see what I may be missing out on.

Compared to med school, business school classes were heaven. The toughest part of the day was deciding whether to go to the Medtronic happy hour or the Mayo Clinic case competition. I became fluent in business jargon, networked my ass off, thought about new aspects of medicine, and made friends with people from a wide variety of work experiences.

People always ask, "How do you use the M.B.A. in your medical career?" When coupled with practical clinical experience gained in residency, the opportunities for a physician with business education are endless: consulting, venture capital, hospital administration, just to name a few. Nonphysician medical leaders take me more seriously—whether or not they actually should. I've also carved out a niche consulting for start-up medical device companies. Finally, my business training is probably why I offer lavender aromatherapy and music to my patients prior to their spine injections. No matter what else happens in my career from a business perspective, I know that my joint degree has made me a much happier and more effective physician.

ROY BRYAN, JR., M.D., M.B.A.
MEDICAL AND BUSINESS SCHOOL: University of Minnesota, Minneapolis
RESIDENCY: Massachusetts General Hospital, Boston
FELLOWSHIP: University of California, Los Angeles

14.
MEDICINE WARDS

Rounding, Admissions, and Discharge Summaries

Medical specialties can be divided into three main categories: medicine, surgical, and other. "Medicine" includes internal medicine, family practice, pediatrics, and the myriad medical subspecialties, including gastroenterology, cardiology, pulmonology, nephrology, and endocrinology. "Surgical" includes general surgery and all of its offshoots and subspecialties, including urology, otolaryngology (ENT), surgical oncology, and orthopedic surgery. Finally, "other" includes everything else that doesn't fit into the two main groups. This includes anesthesiology, emergency medicine, radiology, pathology, occupational medicine, OB/GYN, and psychiatry.

This division also helpfully describes the experience during clinical rotations. Many of the required rotations and electives are within the purview of internal medicine and its many derivatives. I will describe the general nature of these rotations in this chapter. Surgical and "other" rotations are often quite different and will be described separately.

MORNING ROUNDS

Life as a third- or fourth-year medical student on a medicine rotation involves many, many hours of something that most people have never heard of until they enter medical school: *rounding*. No, this doesn't mean rounding up cattle or drawing circles. Though sometimes rounding in medicine wards can feel like one of these.

Rounding is the process of a physician "making rounds"—walking through the hospital in an organized fashion from patient to patient. In the private practice world, a hospitalist might round on a dozen patients in an hour. She might perform a quick chart review, noting relevant nursing comments, reviewing vital signs, and looking at new lab values and imaging results. Next is a quick stop in the patient's room, explaining how things look based on the chart review, asking about the patient's current condition, and performing a physical exam. During this process, the physician will formulate an idea of how things are going, whether any new diagnoses are present, what changes in treatment need to be made, or if the patient is ready for discharge from the hospital.

While that can all take place in five to ten minutes with a fairly simple case and an experienced physician, the process can seem infinitely longer in an academic medical center, in part because patients are more complicated. Many more people are present for rounds—including attending physicians, fellows, residents, medical students, pharmacists, pharmacy students, nurses, nursing students, and other ancillary staff—and historically much of an attending's teaching points are made for the benefit of all trainees during rounds. All of this can add up to "morning rounds" lasting until lunchtime or well into the afternoon.

If you've ever been a patient or visited a loved one at an academic medical center, you've surely seen this process taking place. All will be quiet in your random corner of the medicine ward, when suddenly a herd of a dozen or more people in white coats of varying lengths and labels descends upon your room. Several may have laptops rolled around on wheels, often called "COWs" (computers on wheels) or some equally cute acronym. There are a lot of young people, with a few gray-haired folks running the show and occasionally putting the youngsters on the spot. The gray-haired folks are the attending physicians and possibly an attending pharmacist or seasoned nurse. The young folks are all likely in some form of medical training.

Sometimes an especially young whippersnapper in a short white coat will nervously pull out a folded paper, clear her throat, and begin a ten-minute dissertation about a nearby patient. She will state the name, age, medical history, current issues, number of hospital days, medications and allergies, and exam findings, with varying degrees of fluidity, mostly depending on whether the speaker is a third- or fourth-year student and the time of year. That student's day is going well if the attending listens patiently, asks a few questions, agrees with the proposed treatment interventions, and moves on—not so well if there are frequent interruptions, fumbling responses, questions about whether the person actually attended the first two years of medical school, and tears. Though we're increasingly in an era of kinder, gentler medical training, I still witnessed all of the above several times during my training.

Not all attending physicians follow such a traditional approach. Some prefer to quickly see all patients in person and then discuss things more thoroughly in a workroom with access to computers with lab values, X-ray images, and phones to make consult requests and confirm orders. Most attendings choose patients with interesting exam findings to highlight a particular piece of the physical exam. Often there is an afternoon teaching session that involves everyone reading a journal article the night before, one student or resident teaching everyone about a medical topic, or a random question-and-answer session.

Some variation of this is how virtually every medicine-based rotation plays out. Obviously, a critical care rotation will mean sicker patients, a smaller patient census for the team, and probably more time spent per patient. On the other hand, a consult service on a gastroenterology elective may involve seeing dozens of patients throughout the hospital and then spending some time in the lab after rounds to observe and possibly assist with colonoscopies and other procedures.

Regardless of the specific rotation, as a medical student you are typically assigned a handful of patients to treat as your own. You are expected to come in early for pre-rounding—coming in sometime when it's still dark outside to wake up your patients, check on how they're doing, write down or print out morning vital signs and labs, and look up any new imaging studies and culture results. You are then supposed to synthesize all of this information, come up with a rough idea of what's going on with the patient and how you want to change treatment accordingly. If you're organized, you will have just enough time to accomplish these tasks, maybe grab some coffee, and join the rest of your team for the actual rounds.

During rounds, each time the team stops at one of your patients, you will formally present your patient as taught in medical school. Residents and attendings are often quite picky about the order in which information is presented, which data are read aloud, and how you organize your assessment and plan. And once in a while you will get some new attending who does it completely differently than all your previous attendings. Guess who has to make changes? Hint: It's not the attending.

Each of your patients will also be assigned to a resident, so you're depended upon to some degree but are still fairly redundant—especially as a third-year student. Nice residents may help you out, filling in gaps in your presentation and maybe even running through your patients before the start of rounds. Others may hang you out to dry while your attending pimps you to death and questions whether you even saw the right patient this morning. As the saying goes, shit rolls downhill, so there's not much you can do about that.

ORDERS, M&Ms, AND CHARTING

Once rounds are done and all the patients on the team census have been discussed, with plans agreed upon by the team, it's time to head back to the workroom to make sure all orders are in and write all of the day's notes. Depending on how long rounds lasted, you may try to attend some informational lecture for a free lunch. Various educational conferences and M&M (morbidity and mortality) sessions may require your attendance before or after rounds.

ANOTHER DOC'S SHOES: SHAKE, RATTLE, AND ROLL

Prior to medical school, I had never heard of a pseudoseizure. It's a weird situation in which a patient looks like they're having a seizure—and in some cases legitimately believes they are having a seizure. But they're not *really* having a seizure. Sometimes any physician can readily identify a pseudoseizure by its lack of characteristic movements or other signs that go along with real seizures. Other times, even a seasoned neurologist has to perform extensive studies to distinguish the two.

Some patients fake seizures on purpose, usually for material gain like getting out of work or getting drug injections. However, it is also possible for patients to actually "black out" during a pseudoseizure and really believe they are having seizures—but in reality their minds are subconsciously fooling them. Analysis of brain waves by EEG is usually needed to tell the difference.

One of my first experiences with pseudoseizures was during med school. I was rounding with my internal medicine team when we came across a woman thrashing around on the floor in the middle of the hallway. Her limbs were violently shaking, she was drooling, and her eyes were rolled back in her head. My senior resident appeared to recognize the patient and said, "It's a pseudoseizure. Get some Narcan for intramuscular injection." The patient immediately stopped shaking, and she said, "No Narcan!" Seconds later, she was again shaking with eyes rolled back in her head. Narcan is used to reverse the effects of opiate drugs like heroin and morphine. In an addict, it can induce horrible withdrawal symptoms. Needless to say, seconds after a nurse approached the woman with a needle, her seizure stopped.

"CHRISTINE," M.D.
MEDICAL SCHOOL: Duke University, Durham, North Carolina
RESIDENCY: Northwestern University, Chicago, Illinois

M&Ms have nothing to do with candy; they are (usually) weekly meetings requiring the attendance of all internal medicine attendings, fellows, residents, and medical students. The chief resident presents patients from the hospital who have recently suffered morbidity (injury) or mortality (death), to review relevant medical knowledge and learn from any mistakes made in the patients' care. Traditionally, the residents and students involved often received relentless questioning from attendings and more senior residents and were singled out for lack of knowledge or questionable decisions and actions. Thankfully, a more educational and less punitive approach has gained popularity over the last couple of decades.

Once all the educational stuff is out of the way, you'll have to finish your notes. When you thought about going to medical school, you probably severely underestimated how much time you would spend at a computer writing notes. Charting is the bane of all medical hospital staff. "If it isn't charted, it didn't happen," so everyone says. More important, if you don't chart it, the coders can't bill patients for it. Then nobody's happy.

Although many private practice docs are still working with paper charts, most large academic medical centers now have electronic medical record (EMR) systems. And thanks to government regulations, most every provider will eventually have some form of EMR. This has the benefit of allowing everyone to read chart notes instead of having to decipher the chicken scratch and slew of acronyms that used to populate paper charts. But it also means an explosion of data that are blown into notes, often optimized for billing purposes and not always helpful when you're actually trying to read notes and figure out what's going on with a patient.

For medical students, this means a lot of time laboriously typing notes. Being a speedy typist is a more useful skill in medical school than you may have suspected! Progress notes are the easiest to type. Progress notes include a brief summary of the subjective (what the patient tells you) and objective (vital signs, labs, imaging) events of the last twenty-four hours, as well as a synopsis of your team's current assessment (the patient's issues in terms of formal, medical diagnoses) and plan (what you are doing about each of the patient's issues, in terms of medications, procedures, or consults). So-called SOAP notes (*s*ubjective, *o*bjective, *a*ssessment, *p*lan) don't change much day to day and can be hammered out pretty quickly once you get the hang of it. Just make sure you pay attention during rounds so you remember exactly what your attending and the rest of the team want to do with your patient.

Much more laborious is the admission history and physical (H&P), the initial document written by a physician that describes everything relevant to a patient's hospital admission. This is what you will write when your team is admitting new patients and you are assigned a new patient coming in from the emergency room or who is a consult from another service. Eventually you will learn to quickly get the information you need by reviewing the patient's chart, interviewing the patient, performing a focused physical exam, and ordering relevant labs and imaging studies. You will expertly describe why the patient came to the hospital, their hospital course, subjective and objective findings, and your initial assessment and plan.

Until then, you will spend an hour or more on these behemoth documents, while your residents quickly crank out the same information, enter orders, and move on to the next patient. Don't worry; it's a learning curve. Nobody expects your notes to be perfect. In fact, they don't even officially count for anything and must be cosigned by a resident or attending. And yes, your efficiency will improve.

Once, as a fourth-year medical student, I admitted a patient to an ICU service. The patient was rushed to the operating room, and I spent much of the next hour working on the admission H&P. Before I finished, I was informed by one of the surgical residents that, sadly, the patient had died in the OR. Though I had seen the patient only long enough to perform a quick physical exam and place an arterial line, I of course felt horrible. Yet my sleep-deprived brain did selfishly wonder if I still had to finish the H&P. My resident said yes, it would be good practice.

Finally, there is the discharge summary: a lengthy discourse detailing why a patient entered the hospital, what was done for them, and how things turned out. There's definitely some truth to the old saying that the longer the admission, the shorter the discharge summary. I remember typing detailed discharge summaries for patients who had been in the hospital only a few days, because every last thought and discussion our team had was fresh in my mind.

By contrast, the discharge summary for the patient our team inherited from the prior team, who had been hospitalized for almost two months—with multiple rounds of antibiotics, numerous consults, and several trips to the OR—would get a discharge summary that was half as long. Why? Because all you can say is that the patient came in for something, a whole lot of other things happened in between, and now this is where we're at. When an admission gets complicated enough, nobody sweats the details of the discharge summary. It's obvious that the patient had an unfortunate, complicated hospital course, and the big picture is really all anyone cares about.

In reality, a discharge summary should be a nice, tidy note written by the hospital team that briefly summarizes what happened in the hospital for the benefit of the patient's primary care provider and other specialist consultants. Once you're an attending—and even an experienced resident—this is what your discharge summaries will look like. The same goes for your admission H&Ps and progress notes. They won't be novels. You won't have the time, and nobody else will have the time to read them.

But as a medical student, your job is to learn how things work. You're there to think about all the possible diagnoses that could be involved—even if they're not that likely—and all the treatment options you could provide. You're supposed to secure a really strong grasp of how a patient's hospital course transpired and what events led to complications, lengthening of stay, or improvement in the patient's status.

Much like math class, where you're always reminded to show your work, the directive to medical students to write out every last detail and thought process in medical notes is proof to your superiors—and evaluators—that you do have a good understanding of what's going on and are making good clinical decisions based on the information at hand. Nobody's a mind reader, and if you just jot down the bare essentials, it would be impossible to evaluate what you're learning.

So while charting and writing notes may seem like a real drag while you're a medical student, particularly on medicine rotations where it is often a central component, know that it is only temporary and intended mostly for the sake of learning. You have to know how to write block letters before you can write the traditional cursive, in other words.

If you go into private practice, you will likely have physician assistants or nurse practitioners who help out with your daily documentation. I know a few folks in such positions who see dozens of patients each day and simply tell their ancillary staff the main points that need to be documented, leaving the details to those writing the notes. Of course, if you go into academic medicine, you will have scores of medical students, residents, and fellows to do your bidding.

15.

SURGERY AND THE OR

Life as a Sleepless Human Retractor

If rounding and typing notes are the key features of medicine rotations, the operating room (OR) is the centerpiece of surgical rotations. To be sure, during surgical rotations, you will still round on patients each day and type some notes. But a much larger percentage of your time will be spent in the OR preparing for and assisting with procedures. There is also some requisite clinic time, when you will see patients in an outpatient setting, evaluating them for potential surgical intervention and following their progress postoperatively. In short, the surgical rotation is a vignette of the life of an actual, practicing surgeon.

SURGICAL ROUNDS

For the third- or fourth-year medical student on a surgical rotation, the day starts early—I mean *really* early. It's still pitch black out when you drive to work, and most of the stoplights are still blinking. You will typically arrive a bit earlier than your residents to pre-round on your team's inpatients. Just as with medicine rotations, this involves quickly gathering overnight events, labs, and vital signs, as well as (frequently) waking up patients to ask them how they're doing and perform a brief physical exam. Before you get too upset about waking up before your residents, realize that they were likely up half the night responding to nursing calls and going to the emergency room for consults.

Once your residents arrive, the entire team will quickly round on all inpatients. The process is much the same as on medicine rotations, only the time is more compressed. On surgical rotations, rounding is not the focus of the day, but rather a necessary evil done before and after time in the OR. To be sure, every patient is examined by a resident and attending, and every effort is taken to provide optimal care. But a surgical team just doesn't have the time to spend several hours each day rounding on patients and hashing out the details of differential diagnoses and treatment plans. Furthermore, the bulk of teaching to residents and students on surgical rotations is performed in the OR during procedures, or occasionally during lectures, M&M conferences, or journal clubs held during the morning or afternoon.

Surgical rounds are much more focused and to the point than their medical counterparts, which can be a little disconcerting at first if your initial experiences during the clinical years are on medicine rotations. But the purpose is a bit different. In most cases, the surgical team is focused on the surgical issues. For example, if a knee is replaced, rounds will focus on how the wound is healing, whether the patient is doing well in physical therapy, and the basic clinical issues of input and output, vital signs, and lab values. If a patient has preexisting medical conditions or develops any that are beyond the purview of the primary surgical team, a consult is made to the relevant medical specialty, who will see the patient and manage that specific medical issue.

In addition to examining patients, placing orders, and managing discharges, surgical rounds also can include small procedures, such as changing dressings, cleaning wounds, and removing chest tubes or drains. These tasks are typically performed by residents, but experienced students may share in the bounty if time permits for proper teaching. If you're lucky, you'll rotate through a vascular surgery service and experience the joy of removing a foot dressing from a patient with an auto-amputated toe! Yes, auto-amputation is a thing, and you will eventually know what it is if you don't already.

Writing notes is a necessary evil even during surgical rotations. But again, this is not the focus of a surgical rotation as in medical rotations. You will type brief notes on your patients, quickly summarizing overnight events, relevant vital signs and labs, and an assessment and plan related to surgical and important medical issues. Emphasis is also placed on how many days have passed since the patient's surgery (the "postoperative day" or POD, with POD#0 indicating the day of surgery), which lines or drains can be removed, and whether the patient can be discharged.

On your surgical rotations, you'll learn to move quickly in the mornings, because case start times in the OR dictate the schedule, and you will need to move on when the time comes, whether or not you have finished your notes. Trust me, your overall experience and rapport with residents and attendings will be greatly improved if you learn to finish your notes by the end of your blitzkrieg rounds.

INTO THE OPERATING ROOM!

Your first time in the OR environment can be intimidating, because it's a new environment with a lot of rules and conventions, and nurses who are convinced your primary goal is to contaminate sterile fields. If you're lucky, a helpful senior student or resident will guide you through the basics of finding the locker room, getting scrubs, putting on hats and masks, and other routine actions required just to set foot in the OR. You should join your resident team prior to procedures to introduce yourself to the patients you will be caring for in the OR.

Once in the actual operating room, the general rule is to not touch anything blue. Not everything blue is sterile, and most things in the OR are blue, so you won't be touching much. But that's all right, because when you're first starting, it's probably best to not touch *anything* unless specifically asked to do so.

As a surgical student, you will be wrapping up notes and other daily duties while the anesthesiology team gets the patient off to sleep. You will come into the room shortly thereafter to help the nurses with patient positioning and prepping. Your best bet is to follow the lead of your resident or a senior student. If you can learn about basic OR patient positioning ahead of time, that's even better.

The attending physician typically rolls in after most of the positioning and prepping is complete. He or she gives everything a quick once-over to make sure it's satisfactory. If you haven't already met your attending, this is probably the best time to introduce yourself, and even better if you can help tie up the back of your surgeon's gown. Again, best to watch someone do it first, as you definitely don't want to contaminate anything.

Once the procedure commences, your attending or resident will tell you where to stand. Sometimes you will be instructed to "scrub in" and stand up close to the patient alongside the attending, resident, and scrub tech. Other times, you will be asked to stand on the sidelines somewhere, perhaps watching a live, televised image of the surgery on one of the OR monitors. Don't take it personally if you're not allowed to scrub in; sometimes there just isn't enough room for everyone to fit. Also, much like a football game or large concert, often the view really is better on TV.

During procedures when you do scrub in with the surgical team, you will sometimes be on your feet for several hours. The surgeon may ask you to hold a retractor (a metal blade with a handle, designed for holding organs and tissues out of the area of action) for much of that time, periodically instructing you to make slight adjustments to the position or angle of the retractor. If you ever start to feel lightheaded, dizzy, or excessively sweaty, you should tell your surgical team right away. Don't wait until you faint and fall face-first into the surgical field! They would much rather you scrub out for a while, sit down, and drink some water. Trust me, your role as a human retractor *is* important, but there is *always* some sort of mechanical contraption that can do the same job. Hospitals without medical students somehow do surgeries every day without major difficulty.

In addition to manhandling retractors, you may also be allowed to cut sutures after the surgeon is finished tying a knot. There is a joke that every knot cut by a medical student is always too short or too long. There's definitely some truth to that, but it usually doesn't matter too much. In general, too long is better than too short, for obvious reasons.

Finally, if you have demonstrated enough familiarity with the procedure and have successfully navigated any pimping questions thrown your way, you might be allowed to practice your sewing and knot tying by helping the resident close skin. It's a good idea to practice basic knot skills early in your surgical rotation—if not a week or two before—as it not only will impress your team but also will likely be the most useful skill you take away from your time in the OR, regardless of your ultimate specialty choice. You should first master instrument tying and two-handed tying, and then work your way up to one-handed tying.

That's really all there is to being a medical student in the OR during a surgical rotation. There's often a sense of mystery and fear among medical students about the OR. But if you read ahead about procedures planned for the next day, study the relevant anatomy, and know the basics of your patients, you'll do fine. Nobody expects you to have memorized every surgical tool by the end of the rotation or to be a master of sewing and knot tying. After all, surgical residencies last for at least five years; it takes a long time to master these skills!

EVALUATIONS AND SPECIALTY CHOICE

The most anyone can hope for when you're a third-year medical student (when most students will do their first surgery rotation) is that you not get in the way or make things more difficult. It's a bonus if you help out every once in a while and at least seem reasonably interested in the subject at hand. Show up on time or a bit early, do what's asked of you, and express some interest in your patients, the procedures, and surgical decision making. Do these things, and your evaluations will be fine.

If you're a gunner who is shooting for honors in everything—or you have a particular interest in pursuing a career in surgery—you can make an even stronger impression by staying late to assist with additional procedures, taking a strong ownership in your patients and knowing them inside and out, and practicing basic suturing skills and relevant anatomy prior to starting the rotation. Beyond that, just study and do well on your rotation exam, and an honors evaluation is completely within your reach.

Most students have a pretty good idea by the start of their third year whether they are interested in pursuing a surgical career. If you are still on the fence by the start of your first surgical rotation, keep an open mind and plan to impress. A good evaluation from your surgical preceptors will go a long way when it comes to the residency match.

If you are still undecided as to your career plans, you will most likely have a surgical career ruled in or ruled out by the end of your first surgical rotation. It either works with your personality and preferred work environment or it doesn't. Some students love the pace and tangible nature of surgical work. Others hate it. Very few seem to be ambivalent.

Your core surgical rotation often involves very long hours. You will typically get up an hour or two before you normally would, be on your feet most of the day, and stay at the hospital well past dinnertime. You may spend ten or twelve hours per day in the OR, scrubbed in the bulk of the time, standing and holding retractors. After being on your feet all day watching other people cut and sew, you may find yourself exhausted and tired of being asked esoteric questions about the natural history of appendicitis.

A negative, visceral response to the long hours, physical demands, and sometimes brusque demeanor of the OR may truly indicate that a career in surgery just isn't for you. But it's important to keep an open mind as much as possible. Remember, for surgical residents and attendings, time in the OR is filled with challenging intraoperative decisions, occasional crisis management, and directing the entire flow of the procedure. As a medical student, you are seeing only a fraction of what is actually occurring.

Consider that being a medical student in the OR can be a lot like watching a NASCAR race on TV—assuming you're not a huge fan and know very little about the sport. It may look like a bunch of cars going around in circles over and over. But try to imagine yourself in the driver's seat, racing on a track, going well over one hundred miles per hour, just inches from neighboring cars. Imagine the mental concentration and physical skill required to successfully navigate the course—and the satisfaction of completing the race. That's getting closer to what a surgeon experiences while performing an operation, which is quite a different experience from that of an observing medical student holding a retractor for two hours.

Remember, too, the many nonsurgical specialties that allow physicians to perform procedures. So if after your surgical rotation you are attracted to the idea of using your hands in your career but don't think a career in surgery is for you, there are other options. Examples include anesthesiology (especially if you enjoyed the OR environment but don't find surgery to be your calling), emergency medicine, OB/GYN, family medicine, interventional cardiology, gastroenterology, and pain medicine.

With that, I'll leave you with a few "rules of surgery" that are most relevant to a rotating medical student in the unforgiving environment of the operating room:

1. Until you know what you're doing, don't touch anything blue.
2. Eat, drink, and pee whenever you have the opportunity.
3. Don't cut anything with scissors unless asked to do so.
4. Don't touch anything that's pulsating.
5. Don't try to BS your way through a surgeon's pimping session.
6. It's okay to say, "I don't know."
7. Excuse yourself if you're feeling faint.
8. Don't piss off the OR staff.
9. Don't cut sutures too short or too long.
10. Don't fuck with the pancreas. *(This one will make sense eventually.)*

16.
USMLE STEP 2 CK

"But I *Really* Want to Be a Dermatologist!"

Step 2 CK (which stands for *clinical knowledge*) of the USMLE is either the second most important standardized exam you will take while you are in medical school, or just another pass/fail exam that ranks somewhere in importance between getting your flu shot and remembering to pay your rent on time. It really depends on how well you performed on the USMLE Step 1, your intended specialty, and the rest of your overall residency application package.

DETAILS AND LOGISTICS

The multistate, uniform USMLE is a four-part exam that starts with Step 1 at the end of the second year of medical school, continues with Step 2 CK (clinical knowledge) and CS (clinical skills) sometime during the last two years of medical school, and wraps up with Step 3 during the intern year or second year of residency. Step 2 CK is another day-long, multiple-choice exam administered at a corporate testing center, just like Step 1. The main difference is that Step 2 CK is more clinically oriented (hence the name "*clinical* knowledge") and relies more on clinical decision making and acumen gained experientially through your clinical rotations than on rote memorization alone.

You will still have to study for Step 2 CK, if only to get a feel for what kind of material is tested and the general format of the exam.

Many of the same question banks and review books available for Step 1 also exist for Step 2 CK. If you liked what you used for Step 1, you may want to stick with the same publishers for Step 2 CK. Indeed, there will be some information that you need to memorize, either because you haven't yet taken all of your core rotations or you're just not as comfortable with some topics.

The big variable is how *much* you'll have to study for Step 2 CK. Received wisdom says students spend two months studying for Step 1, two weeks studying for Step 2 CK, and two days studying for Step 3. That's a bit of an oversimplification, but there is some truth to it for a lot of folks. Again, it depends on your specific situation.

CHANCE FOR REDEMPTION? OR JUST *ANOTHER* EXAM?

If you knocked Step 1 out of the park and got a score that is solidly within the average range of scores for successfully matched residents in your intended specialty (information easily gleaned from the National Resident Matching Program website), then probably you have nothing to worry about and can delay taking Step 2 CK until after the residency match, which takes place in the spring of your fourth year of medical school. You also can pretty diligently subscribe to the "two weeks for Step 2 CK" study model and not stress too much about the exam.

Unfortunately, this won't be the case for all students. If you instead have decided you want to pursue a competitive specialty that requires higher-than-average Step 1 scores, you need to very honestly assess your own Step 1 performance and the rest of your CV. If your Step 1 score is below or barely within the range of average Step 1 scores of successfully matching residents, you'll need to devote some serious time to studying for Step 2 CK and plan on taking it early enough to include it in your residency application materials. That usually means taking it toward the middle or end of your third year of medical school. That also means you probably will not have yet finished your core rotations and may well need to study material that you are not familiar with.

It's not the most enviable position to be in, but if you aren't entirely happy with your Step 1 performance and want to improve your chances of a successful match in your specialty of choice, then knocking Step 2 CK out of the park is your best chance. Since you can't arbitrarily retake the Step 1 exam, doing very well on Step 2 CK could suggest to residency directors reviewing your application that your weaker Step 1 performance was an aberration due to an off day or chance events—not an accurate reflection of your academic performance and potential.

Unfortunately, many residency programs still use your Step 1 score as a pure cutoff when reviewing the plethora of applications. This can mean your awesome Step 2 CK score will still never see the light of day. In these situations, I recommend you arrange "away rotations" at institutions you are specifically interested in, so you can show your face and (hopefully) impress people with your personality, clinical skills, and hard work. If you get to know the faculty personally, they will at least review your application and not throw it away unseen. And if you perform well during the rotation and have an awesome Step 2 CK score on file to make up for a less-than-stellar performance on Step 1, you'll still have a shot.

A caveat: You *have* to be very honest with your self-assessment. Try enlisting a second set of eyes from an honest friend or adviser. If you failed Step 1 and barely passed when you retook the exam, or if you have multiple failed rotations or preclinical classes during medical school, or if you were suspended from medical school for a time due to unprofessional conduct or some other issue—then you need to be honest about your chances of matching in a competitive specialty—even with a good Step 2 CK score and personally knowing the residency director. I say this not to destroy hope, but rather to save you wasted energy and time.

Look carefully at the NRMP website I mentioned earlier. Some of the most competitive specialties have had literally *zero* successfully matching residents with a failed Step 1 attempt, going back a decade or more. Sure, you could be the first person to break the trend with your stellar Step 2 CK score, research experience, and awesome personality. But chances are most of the applicants to such residency programs will have stellar scores on *both* Step 1 and Step 2 CK, multiple publications, *and* at least decent personalities. Why would they pick you when they can pick someone with a better application instead?

I know it sounds harsh, but some of these ultra-competitive specialties have so few spots they need to fill that they have no reason to compromise when it comes to choosing applicants for their rank lists. So unless you have a *really* strong relationship with someone in the position to select you for a residency program, you must be honest with yourself.

If you really think you still have a shot, then you can either apply for only the competitive specialty or simultaneously apply for two specialties (more details on this in chapter 18, "Applying to Residency"). As you can imagine, the second option is a bit painful and adds time and expense to the already time-consuming and expensive residency application process. But at least you'll have a safety net.

On the other hand, if you don't feel confident you have a decent chance of matching in your desired specialty, you need to start considering alternative specialty choices. It's better to give this some deliberate thought and make an informed decision than to haphazardly scramble into some random residency program when you find out that you didn't match.

And that, my friends, is the long and short of USMLE Step 2 CK. Just another brick in the wall . . .

17.
USMLE STEP 2 CS

"It Costs *How* Much to Prove I Speak English?"

If USMLE Step 1 is arguably the *most* important standardized exam you will take as a medical student, then Step 2 CS (clinical skills) is arguably the *least* important. Medical students almost universally agree that this was one of the biggest wastes of time and money during their four years of medical school. Unfortunately, a recent posting on the National Board of Medical Examiners (NBME) website confirms that there are no plans to do away with the exam anytime soon.

Step 2 CS is a standardized exam unlike all other USMLE exams. It is administered throughout the year at only five test centers, currently in Atlanta, Chicago, Houston, Los Angeles, and Philadelphia. Test dates are limited, so you have to find time during your already busy clinical years of medical school to travel to one of these testing centers, where the exam takes about half the day.

STANDARD PRACTICE

At the testing center there's checking in, putting your belongings in a locker, and hearing instructions. You all line up in front of one of several doors down fake clinic hallways. A bell rings and you knock on the doors and enter fake exam rooms, complete with exam tables, "standardized" (fake) patients, and other clinical accoutrements.

The testing centers strive to simulate a real clinical environment, but a hint of unreality always permeates the situation. The "patients" are paid to interact with you for fifteen minutes or so, describing their ailments, answering your questions, and allowing you to examine them, sometimes even throwing in some simulated sounds and physical symptoms.

At a set time, another bell rings, and all examinees return to the hallway. You then have another set period for computer entry of your experience: differential diagnoses, exams and labs you would like to perform, and potential treatments. You are graded on a combination of your freehand computer responses and evaluations from the standardized patients. They will assess your interpersonal skills, basics like whether you washed your hands or greeted them appropriately, and whether you asked specific questions based upon their presented histories. All of this is reviewed by exam officials, and you are given a pass/fail score.

DON'T SWEAT IT!

Virtually every American medical student passes this exam. No one I knew in my class had to retake it. Rumor is that the exam was designed in response to increasing numbers of IMGs who came to the United States during the latter half of the twentieth century to practice medicine. Patients and licensing officials found that many of them were clinically competent and easily passing their written exams but had very limited English skills or such a thick accent that they could not be easily understood by average American patients. In response, Step 2 CS was created as a final check to make sure that all licensed physicians in the United States not only are proficient in medical and clinical knowledge but also can speak easily understood English and interact with patients reasonably and professionally.

ANOTHER DOC'S SHOES: FUN WITH FAKE PATIENTS

To help us prepare for real clinical practice and the USMLE Step 2 Clinical Skills exam, my medical school (like many across the country) required us to participate in periodic experiences with so-called standardized patients several times each year. These were basically people who usually pretended to have some sort of disease or ailment, but in some cases they were there simply to allow us to practice physical exam skills that for reasons of privacy couldn't easily be done on other students. Breast, pelvic, and prostate exams are the obvious examples.

I am forever grateful to the many standardized patients I worked with during my med school years. They got paid a modest stipend, but seriously, can you imagine a couple of dozen shaky med student hands sticking otoscopes into your ears all day—or worse? Sometimes working with these patients was entertaining and required a bit of pretend play. The patients were armed with a variety of tricks to emulate real medical conditions, such as vocalizing a fake wheezing sound when a student listens to the lungs. One time a patient with a pretend history of heavy smoking and shortness of breath was faking just such a wheeze, only they must have not noticed when I removed my stethoscope from their back. They finally stopped making the strange-sounding "wheeze" when I cleared my throat and asked how often they smoked.

"JENNIFER," M.D.
MEDICAL SCHOOL: The Ohio State University, Columbus
RESIDENCY: University of Wisconsin, Madison

Whatever the actual purpose of the Step 2 CS exam, all medical students must take it and will likely spend over a grand to register for the exam and pay for airfare and hotel expenses. Again, the pass rate is quite high, especially if you are proficient in English, remember the basics like washing your hands and introducing yourself, and have paid attention during your clinical rotations. Medical schools have also responded to Step 2 CS by incorporating into their curricula so-called OSCEs (objective, structured clinical examinations), complete with standardized patients similar to those found at the Step 2 CS testing sites.

Yes, at some point you will roll your eyes and lament having to waste your time and money on Step 2 CS. But as with much of the medical training process, it's best to just grin and bear it. You certainly shouldn't need to study much for it. Assuming you have gone through some sort of OSCE experience at your med school, you'll likely be more than adequately prepared just by checking out the USMLE online materials that describe the overall flow of the exam day and the possible topics covered.

18.

APPLYING TO RESIDENCY

Black Friday for the Airline Industry

I'm convinced that the increased air travel resulting from medical students traveling to residency interviews between October and February is substantial enough that major airlines have it built into their budgets. Unless you are applying to the least competitive specialties, are sure your application contents exceed the requirements to match into your desired specialty, and have limited your geographic range of interest to a single city, you should be prepared to open up your calendar and checkbook for another expensive, time-consuming phase of medical education—all on top of your normal clinical duties as a fourth-year medical student, of course.

Thankfully, for the most part, the fourth year of med school is academically and clinically less challenging than the third. You are typically done with core rotations by the time applying to residency intensifies. You also have been at the clinical rotation game long enough that it doesn't require as much mental energy. Nonetheless, a massive amount—if not all—of your free time will be consumed by finalizing your specialty choice, narrowing down a geographic region of interest, completing your CV and residency application, traveling far and wide to residency interviews (hopefully), and then stressing out until the infamous Match Day.

THE *CURRICULUM VITAE* (CV)

For those of you with graduate-level academic backgrounds, the term *curriculum vitae* (CV) will be familiar. But for most folks, it's not a commonly used phrase. Like many things in medicine, it's essentially a normal, everyday word translated into Latin. Literally translated, it means "courses of life." Practically speaking, it's a resume style often used in academia, including academic medicine, that by extension is used throughout the medical profession, even after training when applying to private practice positions with no direct connection to academics.

So, yes, it's basically a fancy way of saying resume—or résumé, if you prefer diacritical marks.

It's good to start developing your CV early in your medical school career. There are plenty of helpful online and print resources, and your med school likely has staff whose duties include helping students with CVs and other residency application details. Get the framework down, save the file (and back it up), then just add new items as they come along—that's much easier than having to look back through several years to try to re-create your entire professional history.

There are entire books and websites devoted to CVs; in general, it's much like a resume—with your name, educational pedigree, work experience, and scholarships and awards—but also includes specific features such as licensure information, board certifications, and your academic presentations and publications.

If your goal is to someday become a bona fide academic physician, you will likely maintain a formal CV with literally every last poster presentation, speech, and publication you have ever been involved with in the medical profession. Accomplished medical faculty have hundreds of publications on their CVs, often taking up several pages. In my experience, private practice physicians don't have the time or interest to read such lengthy CVs, so if after training you apply mostly to private practice groups, an abbreviated CV—three or four pages, max—is probably better.

When applying to residency, you should include in your CV everything and anything you think makes you a better candidate. This includes nonmedical work and educational experience prior to or during medical school and presentations and publications of scientific or medical topics that may be outside your desired specialty. Everyone knows first- and second-year medical students are still figuring out their career paths, so nobody will fault you for being first author on some neurology paper when you are now applying to emergency medicine.

You will likely be asked to explain your research and maybe your path from one field of interest to another. That's fine unless, say, you have dozens of publications in dermatology up until the very last minute, then suddenly are applying to pediatrics. Not that you shouldn't still include that information, but you might have to explain, as people will suspect you are either applying to both specialties simultaneously (using pediatrics as your backup) or made a sudden change because you realized you aren't competitive enough for dermatology.

OVERVIEW AND TIMELINES

As with your CV, there are also countless books and websites to assist you with the residency application process. Since the dates and specifics change from year to year, I'm only going to cover generalities here. I recommend visiting the AAMC and ERAS websites for official information and dates, as well as links to other resources. As always, check with your med school to see if there is a staffer who helps students through this very complicated process. You're paying a fortune to get your degree; you might as well take full advantage of the offered services.

In general, you should have a good idea of your intended specialty by late winter or early spring of your third year of med school. I know this seems early, as you will likely only be halfway through your core rotations by this point and have had no time for elective rotations. But there's a lot to organize, and the earlier you know at least what you want to do and a general geographic area of interest for your residency search, the easier things will be. Besides, if you decide you want to pursue a very competitive specialty, you will need extra time to acquire some research experience, schedule away rotations, and secure good letters of recommendation. Finally, there are a few specialties (currently including neurosurgery, ophthalmology, and urology—this list changes periodically) with "early matches" that have slightly earlier deadlines.

Just as with applying to medical school, you will need to take care of some details early on, as they tend to take longer than anticipated. This includes getting letters of recommendation and securing transcripts and diplomas. At some point, you will also likely have to meet with some administrator from your school regarding the crafting of your so-called dean's letter—a fairly standardized letter used by medical schools to summarize students' academic performances for review by residency admissions committees. In it, your school will allude to your class rank in ambiguous terms and mention notable achievements, awards, positive attributes, and red flags.

As discussed in chapter 3 ("Med School Flavors"), the osteopathic and allopathic residency organizations are in the process of merging. As such, I will describe the general timeline for the M.D. (allopathic) residency programs, since that is what I am most familiar with—and will likely be the only pathway by the time you're doing this stuff. Also, I will leave it to you to read about the details of early and alternative match services used by some specialties, such as the San Francisco Match. All the match services have websites.

Sometime around the spring of your third year of med school, you will gain access to this wonderful tool called ERAS (Electronic Residency Application Service), which is run by the National Residency Match Program (NRMP). This is very similar to the online, centralized application process for applying to medical school, AMCAS (American Medical College Application Service). You will enter a bunch of personal information, upload your CV and personal statement (yes, there's another personal statement involved), and enter contact information of your references so they can upload letters of recommendation, which will remain concealed from you.

In the fall of your fourth year, you start the fun part of choosing all the programs you want to apply to! You can search by specialty and geographic regions, display the list of available programs, and check off the ones you want to apply to. Now it might seem like you should just go ahead and apply everywhere, but of course that comes with a cost. There is a one-time fee just to start the ERAS process. That initial fee (around $100) includes a set number of residency programs (currently ten). Each additional program you apply to costs more money. This is designed to prevent people from using a shotgun approach to apply to every program in the country.

You can apply to multiple specialties if you want, and you can include separate personal statements for each specialty. As someone who interviewed residency applicants as a chief resident in my program, I can tell you that if you're going to multitask like this, be sure to select the appropriate personal statement in ERAS for each program you are applying to!

I interviewed one applicant for our anesthesiology residency program who had gobs of research and extracurricular involvement in orthopedics. When I asked him if he was concurrently applying to orthopedic surgery and was primarily interested in anesthesia as a backup specialty, he emphatically denied this and said he was no longer interested in orthopedics. Too bad he selected the wrong personal statement to be included in his application packet for our residency program. This well-written essay told me all the wonderful reasons he wanted to be . . . yes, an orthopedic surgeon.

If you are in a committed relationship with another medical student simultaneously applying to residency—typically the result of a relationship formed during your medical school years—the caring folks at NRMP have a nifty feature called the *Couples Match*. This allows two individuals to apply to residency programs as a team, such that both applicants will be considered before interviews are offered and program rank lists are completed. This certainly adds a complicating factor to the residency match, but it beats the alternative of one person in the relationship matching in New York and the other matching in Los Angeles.

RESIDENCY INTERVIEWS

Sometime around mid-fall of your fourth year, residency programs will (hopefully) send you emails or letters inviting you to interview with them. They typically give you a few weeks to decide, so it's not uncommon for applicants to cancel interviews as the season moves forward, once they have interviewed at a sufficient number of places or they have gotten offers from highly desired programs.

Interviews usually run from October through early February—the worst time of the year to travel, due to holiday rushes and meteorological surprises. Nonetheless, each year medical students fill up airports across the land heading to and from residency interviews. It's not uncommon to meet fellow students on the interview trail and then run into them again several weeks later, in a different state.

How accommodating residency programs are to interviewing applicants depends upon the specialty and specific program in consideration. The more competitive the specialty and the more highly desired the residency program (Massachusetts General versus Fargo Community Hospital, for example—no offense, Fargo), the less the residency program will offer to the applicants.

Otolaryngology at a top residency program? Applicants can expect to get a couple of interview dates to choose from, with little or no flexibility if the student already has prior commitments on those dates. Similarly, the program isn't likely to pay for a hotel room and almost assuredly will not pay for travel expenses. The applicants will be lucky to get a nice dinner the night before and lunch on the interview day.

By contrast, I encountered some of my highly qualified classmates who interviewed at family medicine residency programs in rural Minnesota who had travel expenses and hotel covered, along with the flexibility to pretty much tell the program director when they could conveniently come up and interview. It's all supply and demand.

Interview day usually involves a bunch of med students dressed in conservatively colored suits, many of them carrying around padfolios and a couple of pens. There are sometimes morning and afternoon sessions, so you might have to wait if you're in the afternoon session. Typically breakfast and lunch are served. The chair, program director, or both will give some sort of lecture to applicants about how great their residency program is. Somebody will go over scheduling, curriculum, call, and other such details. Then applicants will disperse to individual interviews with faculty, administrators, and possibly a current resident or two.

Regardless of the specialty, most of my classmates reported interviews to be pretty relaxed, especially compared to medical school interviews. Most questions focus on how students came to the decision to pursue a specific specialty, what brings them to specific geographic areas and programs, what they want to do in their careers, and other general questions to get to know them better as a person. Clinical curveball questions or random "gotcha" interview questions are rare.

Most students leave their interviews with little idea of how they compare with other applicants. If you make it to the point of interviewing, you at least have a shot. They don't waste time on people they wouldn't at all want in their program. And half the time they've already spoken with so many people they hardly remember any details like Step 1 scores or publications. So congenial applicants often leave feeling pretty good about their interviews if they got along well with everyone.

However, the numbers have a way of creeping back into the equation once the residency admissions committee meets at the end of the interview process to rank all the applicants. A horrible personality can make a top Step 1 score irrelevant. But a wonderful personality and great sense of humor will help only so much if an applicant's Step 1 score and academic record are toward the bottom of the barrel within a program's applicant pool.

RANK LISTS AND THE RESIDENCY MATCH

After careful deliberation, each program will submit a "rank list" to the ERAS program sometime in the late winter. Around then, residency applicants have to submit their final rank lists of desired residency programs.

That's when the magic starts! The "residency match" is performed by an ERAS computer algorithm that matches the rank lists of applicants and programs, resulting in a final "match list" sometime in mid-March. This list, in one fell swoop, determines where every medical student in the country will spend the next several years of his or her life.

Carefully read all the instructions on the NRMP and ERAS websites about how to navigate the residency match. I've heard horror stories of applicants making simple mistakes that completely change their match outcomes—particularly applicants who have to apply to transitional or preliminary intern years prior to their main residency. (I'll explain the confusing terminology of internship and residency in chapter 21.)

I emphasize one specific point about the details of the match: the ERAS algorithm runs through the *applicants'* rank lists first, matching programs to applicants and not the other way around. It takes a bit of mental gymnastics to go through examples of this to see how the mechanism would be different if the algorithm ran through each residency program's rank list first, but I encourage you to run through it in your own mind a few times to better understand it. In any event, trust me: you should *rank programs precisely in your preferred order.* Do *not* attempt to outfox the system by trying to predict which programs are ranking you more highly or any other convoluted approaches you may want to try. Rank lists are due sometime in late February. The ERAS computer does its magic, and the results are subject to a final review. By mid-March, the ERAS program tells program directors if their programs "filled" all of their spots. Around then, applicants are told whether (but not where) they "matched" into a residency position.

The NRMP offers a high-tech option to deal with unmatched applicants and unfilled programs, one that didn't exist when I was a student: a new system called the Supplemental Offer and Acceptance Program, or SOAP (it has nothing to do with SOAP notes), basically a smaller, nimbler version of the main residency match. It allows programs and unmatched applicants to create new rank lists based on all available information within a matter of days—instead of weeks, as with the main match. By the end of a week, SOAP works its magic, and most of the unmatched applicants now have *somewhere* to go when they graduate from medical school. Usually a handful of residency positions still go unfilled, but that's a calculated decision on the part of program directors.

Once rank lists are in and the SOAP process is complete, only a few days remain until one of the most discussed, ballyhooed, and infamous of medical school traditions: *Match Day*.

19.
MATCH DAY

Beginning of the End

Match Day is the annual event when medical students across the country finally discover where they're going for residency. This information is distributed in a variety of ways, depending on traditions and institutional preferences. Some medical schools host an informal breakfast or brunch and offer a few cheery and nostalgic speeches; then students privately find envelopes with their names on them, containing the match results.

Other programs are a bit more formal, with more public humiliation. I know of several programs that randomly call students' names drawn from a bowl, forcing each student to open his or her envelope and read aloud their match results for the first time on stage, in front of all their colleagues and families. The last student called to the stage sometimes gets a prize consisting of money or a meal at a fancy restaurant. You couldn't make up some of this stuff if you tried.

Match Day is a mixed bag of emotions at any medical school. Some students don't match at all—certainly a worst-case scenario. These students are now responsible for paying back student loans previously in forbearance but essentially waste a year because they cannot start residency. Thankfully, this is very rare indeed, but it does happen.

Less unfortunate but still justifiably disappointed are students who matched, but not in their desired specialties. On Match Day they learn that their "backup" specialties are now their actual specialties—for the rest of their lives. Most learn to love their backup careers as much as their desired careers. And in many cases, their desired careers probably weren't as perfect and glamorous as they imagined. Nonetheless, their Match Day is not a day of celebration.

Other students match in their desired specialties—just not very high on their rank lists. They find out they will be going to Fargo Community Medical Clinic instead of Massachusetts General. But at least they'll be doing what they wanted to do, so typically these students grin and bear it and celebrate with the best of them.

Finally, there are the lucky ones who not only matched in their desired specialties, but also matched to one of their top—or their very top-ranked—residency programs. Thankfully, most American medical students applying to specialties for which they are reasonably competitive do match to one of their top three picks. The same cannot be said for those coming from international schools, particularly Caribbean programs—or for those students reaching a bit too high with their specialty choice.

Most medical schools have some student-organized post-match celebratory activities. And for most, it is a day of celebration. But even for those who successfully match, there are always bittersweet emotions. Match Day marks the beginning of the end. It's common for many students to match with residency programs far away from their medical schools. In just a few months, many of your closest friends and the people with whom you have spent countless hours studying, dissecting, learning, discovering, and commiserating will be moving to far-flung corners of the country.

By Match Day most fourth-year med students are done with all of their core rotations and most important electives. For most students, the last few months of med school are the calm before the storm. It's a time to learn as much as you possibly can about your new specialty and about being a doctor—with less emphasis on grades, standardized exams, and evaluations. Honestly, none of that really matters anymore. This is the last chance to take advantage of the vast resources available to you as a medical student—your patients, your colleagues, and your residents and attendings—all in an environment in which you have little if any real responsibility. Those days will soon be gone. Intern year is fast approaching!

20.
GRADUATION

Now You're *Really* a Doctor (Almost)

The only ceremony in medical school that trumps Match Day in its nostalgia, emotion, and pomp is Graduation Day. And with good reason—this day marks the culmination of some of the most challenging, exciting, wonderful, and taxing years of your life. Much like the four years that precede it, Graduation Day is filled with mixed emotions. Everyone is ecstatic to have made it through one of the most difficult and intense graduate degree programs in the country—yet all are acutely aware that this day marks the end of a personal era. Friends and colleagues are moving away, new challenges await in residency, and an entirely new level of responsibility looms ahead.

POMP AND CIRCUMSTANCE

Med school graduation ceremonies are like most academic graduation ceremonies—but with an appropriately higher level of reverence and sense of accomplishment in the air. Enjoy your med school graduation— revel in all the pride, excitement, and sentiment. After attending my own graduation ceremonies for both residency and fellowship, I can tell you that your med school graduation is likely the last one you will experience that has the same collegial and nostalgic feel that you had when graduating from college. Not to say subsequent graduation ceremonies are chump change. They are poignant and exciting in their own right.

They're just . . . different. And from colleagues and friends I've spoken with, this is true whether you are graduating from an ophthalmology residency class of two people or an internal medicine class of twenty-two.

LOOKING AHEAD TO RESIDENCY

Now the heaviness of change and new responsibilities comes to the fore. Most students suddenly get really busy with tasks like finding new housing, packing up furniture, and securing moving arrangements. There are always a few springtime weddings, in which your classmates who somehow fostered relationships during the whirlwind of medical school decide to tie the knot before embarking on the new adventure of residency. Sometimes the weddings are of two of your classmates, whom you watched merge into a couple over the four years.

Most medical schools end fourth-year rotations in May or early June. Conveniently, most residency programs start intern rotations on or around July 1, often with a few days of orientation required in late June. If you're lucky, you'll have at least two or three weeks completely free of educational or clinical obligations between medical school and residency.

Of course, there is much to do during this time—especially if you face the common challenge of moving to a new city for residency. You have to find a new home, pack and move, fill out paperwork for your new residency, and take care of the basics including insurance, new physicians, and transferring utilities. If you bought a house during or before med school and have to move somewhere else, there's that to deal with.

It's easy to get bogged down in all of this and feel like you need to hunker down and start studying for residency and continue your lifelong pattern of responsibility and sacrifice. But I urge you: take full advantage of whatever time you have off between med school and residency!

Not everyone can pull this off, for a variety of reasons, but as an example, my wife and I took a twenty-day trip to Tanzania, where we climbed Mount Kilimanjaro and went on safari in the Serengeti and Ngorongoro Crater. And that was while my wife was recently pregnant with our first child and we dealt with the necessities of moving to a new city for residency.

Trust me: you will *not* have such luxury of time and freedom of responsibilities and obligations for several more years!

Whatever you do, please, for the love of all that is holy, do *not* think it will be a great idea to work for those few weeks to save up some money or anything foolish like that. Do not spend your time reading books to prepare yourself for residency. Do not volunteer on a medical missionary trip. Do not spend any time in or within five hundred feet of a hospital or clinic. Do not practice your physical exam skills on your significant other—unless, of course, that's your idea of foreplay. Do not study for USMLE Step 3.

Just slow down as much as you can amid the chaos of starting a new job, maybe moving to a new city, and settling into your new role as a resident. Enjoy your life for at least a few days. Smell the roses. Appreciate the blue sky.

You have no idea what kind of torture awaits you. You only *think* you know what it's like to go thirty hours without seeing the outside of a hospital. Enjoy your free time now, because in the next few years, you will spend more hours inside a hospital than you ever thought possible. You will fall asleep in the most random places because you haven't had a full night's sleep in weeks. Entire movie trilogies will take the world by storm without your knowledge. Musicians will rise in the charts and die of a drug overdose before you've even heard one of their songs. You will no longer think it's strange that it's dark out when you leave for work and go home at night . . . in the middle of summer.

Congratulations! You're about to start residency!

PART III

RESIDENCY AND FELLOWSHIP

21.
TRICKY TERMINOLOGY

The Confusing Language of Residency

There is always confusion among the general public—and even among medical students—about the various terms associated with medical training. The title *medical student* is obvious to most people. That's somebody who is done with college and is attending medical school with the goal of earning a medical degree. Easy enough.

But what exactly is a *resident*? And how does that differ from an *intern*?

In a nutshell, internship and residency are the parts of medical training that come between medical school and practicing as a bona fide attending physician. There is an optional *fellowship* period that some physicians take part in after residency, but I'll talk more about that later.

RESIDENTS AND INTERNS

Many moons ago, residency was so named because young physicians-in-training literally were *residents* at their training hospital. They had small apartments in the hospital and lived there for several years. Nowadays, residents don't live in the hospital, but they still spend upward of eighty hours per week at the hospital, with many nights and weekends spent in dingy call rooms. Residents spend many more hours at home studying for exams and learning their chosen specialties. Since residency takes place *after* graduation from medical school, these years are often called *post-graduate years* (PGY). Using this same nomenclature, residents are referred to as PGY-1, PGY-2, and so on, based on the number of years of residency completed. For example, a third-year resident is called a PGY-3.

Historically, the intern year was the first year of post-graduate training performed by a new physician. Graduating medical students would first match with a hospital for their intern year, and then later during the internship would secure a residency position to complete their medical training and specialization. In those days, the intern year and post-internship residency training were frequently performed at different hospitals. Nowadays, the intern year is typically part and parcel of the overall residency. It's literally just the first year of residency—the PGY-1 year. Most medical students apply only to single residency programs, and wherever they match is where they will spend the entirety of their residency—with a few exceptions.

Mostly for historical reasons, a handful of specialties still have intern years that are completely separate from the remainder of residency. Examples include dermatology, radiology, ophthalmology, and sometimes anesthesiology. For example, all med students wanting to specialize in dermatology have to apply not only to dermatology residency programs but also to separate, one-year training programs to fulfill the requirement of an intern year.

TRANSITION AND PRELIMINARY YEARS

What sorts of one-year training programs fulfill the requirement of an intern year? This is where the terms *transition year* and *preliminary year* come into play. Dozens of hospitals around the country have so-called transition years that provide experiential training to new physicians in a variety of medical specialties. These programs typically feature a few months of inpatient duties on medicine or surgery wards, a month or two of ICU work, and various elective months that can include emergency medicine, radiology, family practice, and OB/GYN, among other things.

The second option for graduating students entering specialties requiring a separate intern year, called a *preliminary year*, is a one-year, post-graduate training program hosted by departments of internal medicine, pediatrics, and general surgery. Matching into a preliminary year guarantees absolutely nothing beyond the first year, and preliminary interns frequently train alongside fully fledged residents in the same department. For example, a medical student who matched into radiology might first complete an intern year effectively functioning as a first-year internal medicine resident. Upon completion of that year, that student then immediately starts work as a second-year resident (PGY-2) in his or her radiology residency program.

Transition year programs tend to have more elective time, feature more variety, and are generally considered a more favorable way to spend one's intern year than a preliminary year in internal medicine or general surgery. Compound this with the fact that most of the specialties that require separate intern years are highly competitive, and you get the strange result that transition year programs are historically among the most competitive programs to match into as a graduating medical student. Students matching into some of these programs often have average USMLE Step 1 scores well above 250.

Because of the über-competitiveness of transition year programs, many students successfully match into a residency program for their specialty but do not match into a transition year program. These students instead have to complete a preliminary year in internal medicine, general surgery, or, less commonly, pediatrics.

CATEGORICAL AND ADVANCED

Categorical is a term used in some specialties to differentiate residency programs that include a built-in intern year from those that do not. For example, most anesthesiology residency programs are *categorical* programs, meaning a graduating medical student matches into only the one residency program. The residents spend their first year doing a variety of rotations very similar to a transition year, but under the direction of the anesthesiology department and frequently with a focus on the most pertinent rotations, such as ICU, preoperative clinic, pain clinic, and surgery.

By contrast, a student matching to an anesthesiology residency that does *not* include a built-in intern year is said to match to an *advanced* program instead of a categorical one. I'm not sure, but I've always assumed these programs were named as such because their residents enter the anesthesiology program as *advanced* trainees who already have completed an intern year.

Most specialties are heading away from doing an intern year one place and then entering the main residency program. For example, all newly accredited anesthesiology residency positions must be categorical; they cannot be advanced programs. But exceptions can be expected for many years to come.

Unfortunately, there's one more situation that makes this a bit more complicated. During the residency match process, a student can match into a preliminary intern year but not match into any residency program for their intended specialty. For example, a student applies for dermatology, matches into a preliminary internal medicine year, but does not match into any of the dermatology programs on his rank list.

Another possible scenario exists because many students put one or two preliminary intern year programs on their rank list after all of their desired residency programs. These serve as a complete backup if the student doesn't match into any of her ranked residency programs. The idea is, compared to a completely wasted year doing nothing at all, it is better to spend one year completing a preliminary intern year that will pay some money, allow the student to leave student loans in forbearance, and potentially provide some good letters of recommendation and help the student match into her desired specialty during next year's match.

Neither of these scenarios is ideal; actually both are feared by countless students anxiously awaiting Match Day. Unfortunately, they do happen to graduating medical students every year. In these examples, the residents are said to have completed a preliminary intern year but are not matched into any fully fledged residency program.

A preliminary year completed under these nonmatch situations is sometimes a good way to spend the first year after medical school. If a successful match occurs the following year, no time is wasted, and the intern can move directly into his or her desired residency program. The only hassle might be having to move to a new hospital and potentially a new city.

There is no guarantee that after completing a preliminary intern year a second attempt in the match process will bring better results. Unfortunately, completing multiple preliminary intern years does not add any numbers to your PGY status. The most you can do with a preliminary intern year is complete your PGY-1 year. Once you match to a legitimate residency spot, you can become a PGY-2. But you can't complete five preliminary intern years in surgery, for example, and declare yourself a PGY-5 general surgery resident ready for graduation.

Thankfully, repeated nonmatch scenarios like this are uncommon. But they do happen to dozens of unfortunate medical students each year. Eventually, for better or worse, most people give up on their dream specialties and decide to pursue less competitive specialties for which they are better suited, given their academic backgrounds. I do know of a few cases of such individuals who decided to drop out of traditional medicine altogether, never completing a residency program and instead pursuing alternative career plans.

I hope this clears up some of the confusion around the terms associated with the years of residency and the different types of intern years. After writing this chapter, I'm amazed I ever figured it out myself. If you're still confused, at least try to remember the following key points:

- You're a *doctor* immediately upon graduation from medical school.

- With very few exceptions, all doctors must complete residency to actually practice medicine in the United States.

- Most residents work around eighty hours per week in the hospital and earn around $50,000 per year. Student loans *do* accumulate interest during this time period, but payment can be avoided by entering into *forbearance* until the end of medical training.
- Residents are frequently identified by their current year of residency, called post-graduate year (PGY) since it marks the number of years since graduating from medical school.
- The *intern year* is really just the first year of residency (the PGY-1 year). It is also sometimes called an internship.
- For most specialties, graduating medical students match into only a residency program and not a separate internship.
- For a few specialties, graduating medical students need to match into *both* a main residency program in their desired specialty *and* a one-year internship program.
  - Residency programs that do *not* include an intern year are called *advanced*.
  - Residency programs that *do* include an intern year are called *categorical*.
- One-year internship programs include transition years and preliminary years in internal medicine, general surgery, and sometimes pediatrics.
- Preliminary intern years are also sometimes completed by graduating medical students who don't successfully match into their desired specialties. Completion of a preliminary year does count as completion of the PGY-1 residency year. However, completion of multiple preliminary intern years is essentially useless without matching into a full residency program.

Clear as mud? That's what I thought.

22.
STARTING INTERN YEAR

Shit Just Got Real

The first day of intern year is always a bit scary, regardless of your assigned rotation. For the first time in your young career as a physician, people in the hospital will actually do what you tell them to do. Talk about performance pressure! Gone are the days of med school when you put in a bunch of notes and orders just for practice.

Thankfully, most nurses, pharmacists, and ancillary staff working at teaching hospitals are accustomed to the usual influx of green interns each July. Unless you're working with an equally green pharmacist, your ridiculous prescription of 50 milligrams of sufentanil (instead of sildenafil) to the patient with erectile dysfunction will surely earn you a phone call asking if you *really* meant to order a fatal dose of pain medication instead of Viagra. You'll stammer something about hitting the wrong key or clicking the wrong box, thank her for her attention to detail, and swallow another dose of humble pie.

The logistics of intern year vary depending on which type of intern year you are doing: surgical, medical, transition, or specialty-specific such as an integrated pathology residency. My prior descriptions of day-to-day activities during medical versus surgical clinical rotations for med students are also fairly representative of the intern year—only think longer hours, more direct patient care, and much greater levels of responsibility.

A YEAR OF FIRSTS

You experience many things as a medical student, but it's different when you're the *doctor*—the one making the decisions. As a fully fledged physician, your intern year is filled with firsts. You will have your first overnight call, which means you will get every page from all the nurses taking care of the eighty or so patients on your cross-cover list. You will run your first code on a dying patient. You may witness your first patient death. You will make your first independent clinical decision that saves a patient's life or greatly improves his or her health. You will also be responsible for a bad decision that adversely affects a patient and potentially hastens his or her death.

You will learn from these experiences. You will gain confidence and grow into the position of the ultimate decision maker. You will develop your sixth sense of knowing when patients are close to death and need immediate attention. You will become comfortable with having incomplete information. You will gain an appreciation of the natural progression of common disease processes, such as diabetes and alcoholic cirrhosis, and the complications that may ultimately kill those patients. You will become a master of quickly prioritizing your patients and focusing on the most important medical problems.

At the start of your intern year, you will frantically juggle countless pages from nurses. You will constantly refer to your favorite app or pocket reference book for medication doses and differential diagnoses. You will have to think about the next step while performing CPR on a patient. You will frequently lean on your senior residents, fellows, and attendings for guidance and approval.

During that year, you will at some point wonder if you can continue. You will encounter patients who make you sad and heartbroken. You will encounter patients who disgust you and piss you off. You will encounter patients and families that give you hope and remind you why you wanted to go into medicine in the first place. You will learn to work on far less sleep than you imagined possible. You will become a little more numb to physical deformity, blood, and even death. You will groan when you learn another patient has rolled into the emergency room when you are exhausted and still have several new admissions to process.

BECOMING A DOCTOR

Finally, twelve long months later, you will go in to work for your last day as an intern. You might communicate with one of the new interns for the following year, perhaps to give a final sign-out of the patient census to your successor. He or she will ask silly questions and respond with a hint of trepidation. You will smile, realizing just how far you've come and how much you've learned.

Here's an example from my own internship. I started in the surgical ICU, along with one other intern, a fellow, and two residents who were away at a conference the morning we started. The fellow met us briefly that morning and gave each of us three patients to see before rounds with the attending. It took me forever to pore through the plethora of data accompanying my first patient. I don't think I ever even got to my third patient. I certainly didn't have any time to start working on notes.

My fellow stopped by and told me we would be rounding in just a few minutes. My heart sank as I realized I was nowhere near ready to present the three patients in any meaningful way. Of course I can't remember the details, but looking back, I'm sure my presentation was a colossal waste of time. Thankfully, the fellow had quickly seen all six patients in the time it took me to see two and filled in all the blanks from my shoddy presentation. In the true spirit of medical education, the attending lectured my fellow intern and me on how much information we'd missed, how long-winded and disorganized our presentations were, and how much we needed to improve. Welcome to residency!

By contrast, during my final week of internship, I arrived one morning at the hospital to admit my team's first new patient from the ER—an elderly gentleman with end-stage cancer. His condition was rapidly declining, and it had been days since he was able to eat or drink anything without choking and aspirating the contents into his lungs. He was extraordinarily weak, thin, and malnourished. He had presented overnight with a high fever, abdominal pain, and an elevated white blood count, suggestive of an infection. The overnight team had appropriately ordered intravenous hydration, a series of labs and blood cultures, and imaging studies to look for a possible infectious source.

My senior resident and attending were away at a morning conference, leaving me to tend to our team's patients until their return. I spoke with the patient and his family. He was anxious about undergoing more studies and nervous about the possibility of another surgery. The family was at a loss about how to continue caring for him at home. He was reluctant to accept aggressive hydration or tube feedings, as he didn't want to prolong the inevitable. Considering his diagnosis, his physical appearance, and recent imaging studies demonstrating his worsening disease process, clearly this man was in his final days. He may very well have had an infection, but this was not the pressing issue.

After a long conversation with the family, we agreed it was best to consult a palliative care physician to discuss the next steps in managing this patient's terminal disease. I called my attending physician about my plan, and after reviewing the patient's chart, he agreed and told me to proceed and call with any questions. Later I met in the patient's room with the palliative care team, the patient, and multiple family members. I led the conversation, summarizing the patient's medical diagnosis, current condition, and immediate issues. The palliative physician then led the patient and his family through the next steps of ensuring the patient's final days would be as comfortable as possible.

I called my attending to update him, and he agreed. I canceled all remaining labs and imaging studies, discontinued the aggressive hydration, and allowed comfort feeding as tolerated. I prescribed pain medication and acetaminophen for the fever. That afternoon, our medicine team rounded on the entire census, including my dying patient. He was in his room, enjoying some food, and laughing with his family while they watched a movie on the television. The palliative care team was arranging to have him transferred to a palliative wing of the hospital. The patient and his family were all in agreement and deeply appreciative. My attending said, "Nice work," and we moved on to the next patient.

I tell this story not to toot my own horn, but rather to illustrate what intern year is all about. Sure, you will learn basic medication names and doses, differential diagnoses, and simple procedures. You will become comfortable managing many patients, efficiently and often with incomplete information. You will know when patients are *really* sick and need your urgent intervention—and when they are not so sick and can wait.

But the most important things you will learn are how to quickly assess the overall health of a patient, determine which of their disease processes are primarily driving their current situation, decide what's important and what's not, and recognize when additional treatment is not the answer. These things come with countless weeks and months of experience and exposure to numerous patients with various diseases, all in different stages of the disease processes. That's what intern year is all about. The acquisition of this intuitive sense of life, disease, and death starts during the intern year and creates the foundation for all that you will learn during the remainder of residency.

ANOTHER DOC'S SHOES: COMING TO AMERICA (FROM POLAND)

Coming to the United States for residency after completing medical school in another country presents many challenges, especially adjusting to a different health care system and work flow. It is very helpful to set up elective rotations in the United States during summer or electives months in med school. These are even more helpful if done prior to applying for residency, as the American experience can lead to not only possible interviews but also letters of recommendation.

The actual practice of medicine is not all that different between the United States and Europe. Taking a patient's history, performing a physical exam, and producing a diagnosis and treatment plan are universal. However, a foreign physician may be initially overwhelmed by the amount of information and data, as well as the number of patients. Experience in American hospitals *before* residency can be invaluable, as you will be much more comfortable gathering data on patients using electronic medical records.

Finally, you should be prepared for constant communication about your patients with an endless number of people—something that I think is unique to the American health care system. A large portion of your life as an intern will be spent on the phone relaying information about your patients to fellow physicians, social workers, physical therapists, and so on. At first, you may feel like you are a puppet attached to a million strings. But you will eventually discover that you, the lowly intern, are conducting an entire orchestra of health care providers to give proper care to your patients.

PIOTR RUTKOWSKI, M.D.
MEDICAL SCHOOL: Jagiellonian University Medical College, Krakow, Poland
RESIDENCY: Medical College of Wisconsin, Milwaukee
FELLOWSHIP: University at Buffalo, New York

23.

USMLE STEP 3

Nobody Cares—Really

Let's briefly recap the multiple "steps" of the United States Medical Licensing Exam (USMLE). Step 1 is unquestionably the most important exam you will take during your four years of medical school. Step 2 CK is your chance to maybe make up for less-than-stellar performance on Step 1. Step 2 CS is probably the biggest waste of time and money you will encounter during your four years of medical school.

So what about Step 3?

You've already read the title of this chapter.

It's true. *Nobody cares—really.*

Seriously: Just pass the damn thing. Enough said.

As for the logistics, most people take the exam sometime during their intern year, possibly early in the second year of residency. It's the only USMLE that requires you to spend *two* days at a commercial testing center. The first day is a typical eight-hour affair. The second day wraps up around lunchtime or early afternoon.

Just like the other USMLEs, it's critical to spend at least some time learning about the flow of exam day. This is particularly important for Step 3 because it has one section that's a bit different from the other USMLEs. Toward the end of day two, you will leave the warm and comfortable world of multiple-choice exams. Step 3 features computer-based case simulations designed to test how you independently manage patients during clinical encounters from start to finish.

The simulations take a little getting used to, so I strongly recommend at least taking a look at one of the computer-based study aids—a commercial test preparation product or a free sample on the USMLE website. Get familiar with how these simulations work so you can focus on the clinical decision making and medical knowledge, instead of getting bogged down in the logistics of the simulator software.

In all seriousness, as the *final exam* in the medical licensing sequence, Step 3 is still a challenging exam—the last checkpoint to make sure you are fully prepared to practice general medicine independently. Questions focus on general medical issues, primarily with patients in general clinic, emergency room, medical-surgical ward, and critical care settings. There are few questions about esoteric subspecialties or procedural details.

If you've made it this far and successfully graduated from medical school, completed all other parts of the USMLE sequence, and succeeded in your intern year, you'll do fine on Step 3. Just review general medical knowledge that you may not deal with frequently in your particular internship, and familiarize yourself with the design and flow of Step 3, especially the computer-based case simulations.

Pass the exam. Nobody cares about your score, so just relax and pass the exam.

When you leave the testing center on the second day, odds are very good that you will never have to take another USMLE in your life. And that's a pretty good feeling!

A few weeks later, you will receive your results in an email. If you passed, you have successfully completed the USMLE test sequence and are eligible to apply for medical licensure in your state of practice.

Of course, you'll now discover that acquiring a medical license requires a slew of paperwork and several hundred dollars. But what did you expect?

24.
STARTING RESIDENCY

"Now This Is Really What I Want to Do! Sort of . . ."

The transition from internship to the remainder of your residency is much less dramatic than the transition from medical school to your intern year. Depending on your specialty, the intern year may be so integrated into your overall residency that you'll see no difference from one day to the next. But for more residents, no longer being the most junior physician in the hospital is a momentous achievement.

As a second-year resident, you are the one with experience, the resource interns will go to with questions. They will ask you how to put orders into the electronic medical record system. They will also ask you to look at their patient in the ICU and make sure they aren't missing something. They will show you a patient's overnight vital signs to help them figure out why the labs look so bad this morning. Just a year ago you were the tenderfoot on the hospital wards, the lowest physician on the totem pole; now you are the one with a year of wisdom under your belt.

A WELL-DESERVED PROMOTION

Moving beyond intern year typically means you spend less time on hospital wards tending to the basic, day-to-day needs of inpatients. Depending on your specialty, you will likely spend more time doing what first attracted you to your medical field. In surgical residency, you will spend more time in the operating room, establishing your surgical skills and learning to navigate intraoperative challenges. In medical residencies, you will spend more time in critical care units, outpatient clinics, and medical electives, exploring the various available subspecialties, such as cardiology, pulmonology, and endocrinology.

As an anesthesiology resident, my second year of residency meant spending countless hours in the operating room learning the basics of my craft. Within a few weeks, I was on my own in the room, left with an unconscious patient, a surgeon, nursing and technical staff, and the constant beeping of the pulse oximeter. My attending physician was always a quick call away—but things can change quickly in the OR.

I remember several times waking up in the middle of the night from a dream in which I was still in the OR, glued to the patient's vital signs, suddenly aware that I couldn't hear the comforting tone of the pulse oximeter. A few times I awakened with a jolt, grasping for my wife next to me, thinking she was a patient needing resuscitation. Strange, I know, but such things happen when you're running on fumes of sleep and dealing with sick and dying patients day in and day out. It's all part of the joy of residency.

Most often, the start of post-internship residency is a relief. You receive daily confirmation that you chose an appropriate specialty for your interests, personality, talents, and desired lifestyle. Surgery residents are finally spending most of their time in the operating room. Radiology residents are finally in the reading room. Even internal medicine residents can leave the drudgery of floor management and explore subspecialties of interest and take on more leadership roles in the wards and critical care units. The hours aren't always better, but the work is typically a step up compared to intern year—even though the responsibility is even greater.

SECOND THOUGHTS AND CHANGING SPECIALTIES

Unfortunately, I know a handful of people from my med school class for whom the start of their residency was a rude awakening that this was absolutely *not* what they wanted to do for the rest of their lives. Yes, this does happen, but it's not common. Thankfully, there is usually an available escape hatch. It might cost you a year or two of your life in terms of extra residency years, but a year or two spent in any alternative residency program will benefit your medical knowledge and clinical acumen.

Being an anesthesiologist, I can freely say that my own specialty is a fairly cliché example of an escape hatch for surgical residents—and sometimes practicing surgeons—who no longer feel the call of surgery. The expression "If you love working in the OR, become a surgeon; if you like working in the OR, become an anesthesiologist" isn't all in jest.

I'd slightly modify that, because in reality anesthesiologists actually spend more time in the OR than most surgeons, the latter also being burdened with the necessary evils of managing their floor patients and attending clinics. By contrast, most anesthesiologists work in the OR environment day in and day out with no interruption. Thankfully, I love working in the OR and dealing with surgical patients. I find the immediate results and tangible nature of the OR very satisfying, compared to the more long-term and contemplative pace of most medical specialties.

However, I agree with another truism: To specialize in a surgical field, you need to admit to yourself and truly believe that you will not be happy being anything else in the world except a surgeon. A surgical residency is one of the longest, most life-consuming courses of medical training that one can pursue. As hard and as long as I worked in residency, I will never try to argue that I had it harder than any of my surgical colleagues.

Although there are options after training for somewhat more manageable lifestyles in surgical fields, most surgeons still work long, hard hours in practice. And unlike those in many medical jobs spent mostly seated in an office or walking the hospital floors, some surgeons spend their entire working life standing for hours at a time, forgoing normal bodily functions like eating, drinking, and urinating, and still having to deal with calls in the middle of the night and missing family events in the evening because a surgical case went long.

Yet most surgeons I know love their work—even those who have been in practice for years. And that's as it should be. Nobody should go through all the years of training and then deal with the long hours and highly physical work of a surgical practice to do something they only sort of like.

Thankfully, that's where anesthesiology fits in. Many surgical residents figure out in their first or second years of residency that it's just not worth it for them. Perhaps they still enjoy working in the OR environment with surgical patients, but they are content with a different role. Many of them realize they can use their surgical intern year to fulfill their anesthesiology intern year, transferring to an anesthesiology residency program with only three residency years left. So in the best-case scenario, they may lose absolutely no time doing extra years of residency.

I use the anesthesiology example only because it's something I'm very familiar with—not from personal experience (I was never a surgical resident), but from observation of and discussion with several of my colleagues. There are similar examples through all the medical specialties. I know surgical residents who transferred into radiology, family practice residents who transferred into anesthesiology. Indeed, I also know many practicing physicians who in the midst of their careers decided to start a second residency to change their specialty.

The point is that early in residency, you will most likely sink or swim in your chosen specialty. You might not always feel like you made an excellent choice. I think all physicians question whether they made the right choices at various times in their careers—not just with specialty choice, but the entire decision to become a physician in the first place. But you will know something is wrong if, early in your residency, you consistently have a visceral and overwhelming feeling that you do not belong in your chosen specialty.

ANOTHER DOC'S SHOES: THE OL' SWITCHEROO

During my second year of residency training, I realized that a career in surgery, while exciting and rewarding, was not a good fit for my personal and professional goals. After much soul searching and long discussions with friends and mentors, I decided that radiology was a better specialty for me. This decision was both liberating and terrifying. On the one hand, I finally knew what I wanted to do in medicine. On the other hand, I had no guarantee I could make it happen.

Unlike the med school residency match, there is no formal process for switching residencies in the middle of training. Yet it is not uncommon for young doctors to do just that. I was honest with my program director and, to my surprise, she was incredibly supportive. It seems most physicians understand that specialty choice is an intensely personal decision, and if you are not genuinely excited about your field, you are unlikely to become a passionate, caring doctor. It was refreshing to feel the support of almost all of my surgery colleagues and mentors. I think it helped that I was honest, told them early in the process, and honored my commitment to stay in my surgery program through the end of the year.

Next I had to find a new residency position. There are two ways to do this. You can either reapply through the match (along with fourth-year medical students) or find a position outside of the match. The latter is preferable so you don't have to waste any years of training. I emailed my personal statement and CV to the program director at each residency I was interested in, explaining my situation and inquiring if they had any unexpected openings that they were filling outside of the match. Thankfully, I was offered such a position.

Choosing a specialty is a difficult decision made with limited information and time. While I would never recommend choosing a specialty with the intention of later switching to a different one, it is not uncommon for this to happen to residents. During my radiology training, I encountered many attendings who had started in other fields, and their perspectives often echo mine. I have never regretted my decision and am grateful I had the courage to make the switch.

GEOFFREY RUTLEDGE, M.D.
Medical School: University of Minnesota, Minneapolis
Residency and Fellowship: Massachusetts General Hospital, Boston

Personally, I thoroughly enjoyed the work I did during most of my residency. Only a few rotations weren't among my favorites. However, I often thought "I love what I'm doing, but I wish I wasn't doing so *much* of it." Most residents look forward to a day when having one day off per week isn't the norm and when they are not consistently working twenty-four-hour shifts or thirty hours straight in the midst of eighty-hour workweeks.

Nonetheless, I did encounter several residents who were truly unhappy with their specialty choices. All were able to make changes to find something more compatible. One fellow anesthesiology resident I worked with decided early in his second year of residency that he preferred the work he did during his internal medicine preliminary intern year. Fortunately, he was able to transfer back into that same internal medicine program and complete a three-year internal medicine residency, only "losing" the one year he spent as an anesthesiology resident after his intern year.

IN-SERVICE EXAMS AND PIMPING

For the most part, residency is much more like work than school. Exams are much less frequent, eventually coming down to only one or two in-service training exams per year. These are standardized exams, often taken by all residents in a given specialty on a specific day, that give residency programs a sense of where their residents stand compared to the national average in terms of clinical knowledge expected within the specialty.

The top-scoring resident on in-service exams from each class will sometimes get an award at that year's graduation ceremony. On the flip side, the folks unlucky enough to score within the bottom 10 to 15 percent of national scores are typically required to meet with the program director and perhaps do some additional training or coursework the following year to improve their clinical skills and knowledge. It's essentially remediation, and it's best avoided if at all possible. In short, while nobody really cares about the specific grades earned on in-service exams, there's still some pressure to do well—and most residents do spend much of their free time studying during the few weeks preceding each exam.

The "final exam" of residency is board certification. Some specialties have only written exams; others also have a subsequent oral exam. More on these shortly; in essence, in-service training exams are what residency programs use to make sure residents are constantly adding to their knowledge base and staying on top of their material enough to pass their board exams. No residency program wants to consistently crank out a bunch of residents who struggle to become board certified.

The only other nonclinical tests of knowledge come from daily pimping sessions, which vary in frequency and intensity depending on the attending physician and fellow on service. Recall that *pimping* in medical parlance is the act of someone higher on the medical food chain asking someone lower a series of questions regarding medical knowledge or clinical decision making. After the subordinate trainee squirms and struggles for the correct answer, the superior either explains the answer or instructs the subordinate to review the material and possibly present to the entire team the following day.

So I guess residency is more like work, assuming that your boss stopped by your cube several times per day to ask you a random question about your job, assembling your colleagues to hear your answer.

WHO'S THE BOSS?

Another way residency is unlike most jobs is that your boss (the attending physician) keeps changing, from once a day to once every week or so, depending on your rotation and specialty.

For example, an attending physician typically staffs an internal medicine ward team only one or two weeks at a time. They are often on call the entire duration of that week, but most day-to-day decisions are handled by the various members of the team, starting with the medical students and working up through the interns, senior residents, and possibly fellows. Each works to the top of his or her ability, calling upon more senior members when needed. The buck always stops with the attending, so a week on service can be fairly taxing, and such punishment is usually doled out only a few days at a time for post-training physicians.

I spent most of my anesthesiology residency in the OR, often with a different attending physician each day. Anesthesia attendings typically work with one or two residents per day, depending on the complexity of their cases. Attendings and residents are usually assigned to cases by pairing the individuals' positions in the call schedule with the cases' anticipated length. Since residents and attendings hardly ever have the same call schedule, the pairings are almost always different. This highly variable staffing model is common with anesthesiology residents, and it requires constant adaptation on the part of residents to tailor subtle techniques and plans to the liking of each attending.

That really is the nature of residency, regardless of specialty. Every day you work with a slightly different team. The attending physician always sets the overall tone and medical plan. In his or her absence, the fellow runs the show. Then it's the most senior residents, the junior residents, the interns, and finally the medical students. It always runs downhill in that fashion. As such, medical students have to be the most malleable and go with the mood of the moment. Residents and fellows are somewhere in between. And attendings can pretty much do whatever they want—though throwing surgical instruments and making interns cry is becoming less acceptable in medical culture.

BECOMING YOUR OWN DOCTOR

Thankfully, as you progress through residency, your attendings get to know you and increasingly trust your medical knowledge and judgment. As such, you can increasingly run the show your way. In fact, this is encouraged; it signals to your superiors that you are becoming a real physician and expert in your specialty. It's never good when a senior resident months away from graduating is still waiting for his attending to prescribe every action and is unwilling to make independent decisions.

Your goal as a resident should be to learn from every attending and senior resident or fellow above you. Try out the different techniques; see which ones make sense to you and work best with your overall practice. Gradually, you'll develop your own style, and you'll find your subordinate trainees anticipating your decisions and actions because they know that's how you always do things. You won't even realize you had a way of doing things; it just happens.

Finally, residency always features some special projects. The ACGME is increasingly interested in promoting resident involvement in research projects, quality improvement initiatives, and presentations at conferences and lectures. You can expect requirements to participate in these types of activities throughout residency. Of course, no time will be allotted to completing these tasks, so it usually just comes out of your copious free time—which doesn't actually exist.

That's residency in a nutshell!

You've graduated from learning the basics of patient management during your intern year; now you spend two to six years (depending on your specialty) becoming a master of your craft. You will work long hours, spend many nights at the hospital, come in early and stay late when you don't want to, deal with attendings with all sorts of dysfunctional personalities, complete a smattering of research and quality improvement projects, save some lives, make many mistakes, teach those who don't know as much as you, and learn from those who know more than you—and sometimes those who know less than you, too. Somehow, you will emerge ready to practice independent medicine as an expert in your field. Now you're *really* a *real* doctor!

YOU'RE FIRED

That's how things play out for 99 percent of residents that make it this far in the medical education continuum. Unfortunately, I would be remiss if I didn't tell you about one more possibility that can cause havoc for many years—if not for the remainder of one's career. I didn't realize this until I was already immersed in residency, and I've found many pre-meds and med students equally oblivious. Believe it or not, every year dozens if not hundreds of residents across the country throughout all specialties are *fired* from residency!

Firing a resident is never undertaken lightly by residency program directors and review committees. They know it diminishes resident morale, makes a mess of resident scheduling and hospital staffing, damages the reputation of the residency program, produces a bunch of paperwork, and, perhaps most important, can be detrimental to the dismissed resident.

Imagine this scenario: you struggled through medical school, acquired mountains of debt, are now multiple years into residency—probably with some knowledge that things aren't going well. Suddenly you are dismissed from your residency program and cannot practice in your desired specialty! One resident I knew in this situation ultimately pursued a different career altogether. Another found a different residency program from which he ultimately graduated. Some have to start over in a different specialty—perhaps one for which they are better suited.

Thankfully, resident dismissal is very rare. I could not find any hard numbers on this, presumably because residency programs and the ACGME would rather not publicize it. But it can and does happen. Yet another reminder that simply getting into med school is absolutely no guarantee that you will coast through the rest of medical training and land softly in your dream job as a physician in your specialty of choice.

25.
RELATIONSHIP ADVICE

Residency and Beyond

In my experience, serious relationships that survived the tumultuous years of med school seemed to endure into residency—though a few exceptions do come to mind. By this time, most couples have figured out mechanisms for coping with the busy, erratic schedules and other demands of a medical trainee. It also doesn't hurt that residents are finally starting to bring in money instead of hemorrhaging cash and racking up debt. Still, new challenges frequently confront established couples during these years, including moving to a new city, working even longer and less flexible hours, and possibly starting a family.

Another common theme during residency is that with each passing year, the percentage of residents in a relationship increases. Many of these were born during the final months of med school, while others somehow blossomed within the extreme time constraints of residency. It's not uncommon for residents to start dating each other, though a surprising number find partners outside of medicine.

PACK YOUR BAGS

The first challenge to relationships experienced during residency is simply *starting* residency. For example, one classmate of mine who entered medical school as a mid-career change had been married for decades. I can't speak to what transpired in his relationship during medical school, but the last straw appeared to be his matching into a residency program halfway across the country, where neither he nor his wife had any friends or family. Though having to move for their work isn't unique to residents, the stress of transplanting one's life and family to an unfamiliar place is compounded by the extremes of a resident's life.

Your significant other may have already moved for your career once to follow you to medical school. You might be able to guarantee remaining in the same city if you are pursuing a relatively uncompetitive specialty. But if you are interested in a competitive medical field or are only marginally qualified for your specialty of choice, you will likely have to cast your residency application net across a wide geographic area. And you may have no idea where you are going to match until Match Day, in the spring of your fourth year of med school.

Your significant other will have very little time to mentally or emotionally prepare for the move, possibly to a completely new place with no support network. And the moment you arrive to start your intern year you will be overwhelmed with work and studying. You will spend at least sixty to seventy hours per week at the hospital, and much of your time at home with your nose in a book or sleeping. This can be very challenging for your partner, especially if he or she is also working outside the home or left with the bulk of child care duties—or both.

Financial stressors also arise. Government-issued student loans can be placed in forbearance during medical training, which means payments are not due, but interest continues to accumulate. Students who required additional, private loans may have payments already due during residency. And securing a home loan may be difficult, given the relatively low resident salaries compared to the massive amounts of student debt. The only financial positive during residency is that the resident will likely spend so much time in the hospital that he or she will have very little time to actually spend any money!

SOCIAL SUPPORT FOR SIGNIFICANT OTHERS

Some residency programs offer social groups for residents' partners. My residency program did, and my wife absolutely loved it. She worked for part of my residency, then stayed at home with our small children for the latter half. We had some family nearby, but no pre-existing friends in the city where I attended residency. She developed many close friendships from the group, and in particular enjoyed the camaraderie with others who could relate to the specific challenges that come with being in a relationship with someone in the throes of medical training.

I encourage you to inquire about such a support group when inter-viewing at residency programs if you have a significant other, especially if he or she is not also a resident. Although these groups are often still called "spouses' associations," the organization at my residency, for one, was open to any partners of residents, regardless of marital status, gender, or sexual orientation. If you have any questions about member-ship requirements, ask.

If such a group is not available where you attend residency, look for similar support networks on the Internet. However you accomplish it, helping your significant other find some social support system is critical to happiness for both of you during residency.

DUAL-PHYSICIAN COUPLES

I am not married to another physician, but I know several dual-physician couples, most of whom met during medical school or residency. These couples have the challenges of both individuals being extraordi-narily busy, dedicated to their training, and frequently pulled in different directions by their separate training and career ambitions. Residents have only limited control over their call schedules, so conflicting schedules and night floats are commonplace. From conversations with couples I've known in such situations, it's not uncommon to go days if not weeks spending no more than an hour or two in each other's company.

ANOTHER DOC'S SHOES: MIXING BUSINESS WITH PLEASURE

Dating in med school and residency is inevitable. You spend more time with your classmates than with anyone else. You're surrounded by bright, attractive young people, and sparks are bound to fly during late-night study sessions, post-exam parties, or campus football games. There is a chance you'll find your future spouse in your med school class. There is an even greater chance you'll go on a few dates, have a few hookups, and then break up. Even if you don't end up in holy matrimony, a med school classmate can still create an exciting, memorable chapter in your book of dating. The key is to be kind, gentle, and respectful during the relationship and during the breakup, because there is a good chance you'll need to consult with that person on a challenging patient someday.

P.J. SIMONE, M.D.
MEDICAL SCHOOL AND RESIDENCY: University of Minnesota, Minneapolis

Additional challenges include the Couples Match, discussed previously, and potential conflicts over pursuing additional fellowship training or choosing where to work for one's first post-residency job. I've known couples in which one person was done with residency before the other but wanted to pursue fellowship afterward. The other resident had to find work for one year, then move where the fellowship-bound spouse matched and find yet another job. As you can imagine, lots of not-so-pleasant conversations and compromises are inevitable.

Starting a family while both members of a relationship are in residency brings its own obvious challenges. Having family nearby that can help with child rearing is a huge plus, but it's not always possible. And without additional financial resources, full-time nanny services are typically out of reach for a two-resident couple. Traditional day care is always a challenge, as residents often must be at work before day care centers even open—and frequently don't leave work until after they close. And the option of leaving work to pick up a sick child is not exactly encouraged in residency. I know a handful of couples who managed this while both parties were in residency, but I really have no idea *how*—and I wouldn't wish such a challenge upon my worst enemy.

Having a significant other can be a wonderful asset, providing much-needed support during the mentally, emotionally, and physically taxing years of residency. Yet a relationship can add its own stress when you have very little control over your time and your attention is constantly divided by work and studying. Relationships that survive these challenging years emerge stronger, as both partners are forced to hone their skills of communication and compromise. But it's no walk in the park, and you and your significant other need to be prepared.

26.
SLEEP AND HOBBIES

Apparently *Not* Required for Life

During one of my fellowship interviews, a faculty member asked me, "So, what do you like to do you in your free time?" He was just making small talk, but I couldn't help but laugh.

I replied, "I'm in the middle of my chief resident year, studying for written boards, with a two-year-old and a newborn at home. I can't remember the last time I *had* any free time!"

SLEEP DEPRIVATION

Medical training will test the limits of your ability to maintain interests and activities outside the world of medicine. This includes relationships, family, friendships, exercise, hobbies, sports, and nonmedical reading. Most people can preserve a couple of these things while in medical school and residency, but at least two or three fall by the wayside.

Medical training will also test the limits of your ability to function with very little sleep. My wife can tell dozens of great stories about me falling asleep at parties, standing up, or lying on the ground on a bed of rocks while playing with my extremely loud and boisterous children. A friend of mine in surgical residency once actually fell asleep while he was telling a story at a dinner party. I remember frequently falling asleep on elevator rides at the hospital, while waiting in line at the cafeteria, and at stoplights while driving home.

Perhaps the worst was when I momentarily nodded off with an awkward head-jerk while seated on a metal stool between the legs of a laboring patient in the process of delivering her baby. Don't worry, it was only a half-second of slumber, and the resulting adrenaline rush left me wide awake in time to catch the baby (who was fine). But your body will let you get away with sleep deprivation for only so long before it forcefully thrusts sleep upon you whenever—and wherever—you have even a few seconds of possible shut-eye.

WORK HOUR RESTRICTIONS

Now I'm sure some people reading this will say, "Oh, but aren't there work hour restrictions now? Residency's not *that* bad anymore, right?"

Yes, there *are* work hour restrictions now, but they're still a far cry from a forty-hour workweek. Here's a summary of the work hour restrictions that were put into place by the American Council for Graduate Medical Education (ACGME) in 2003:

1. An eighty-hour weekly limit of clinical work, averaged over 4 weeks, inclusive of all in-house call activities

2. A ten-hour rest period between duty periods and after in-house call

3. A twenty-four-hour limit on continuous duty, with up to six additional hours for continuity of care and educational activities

4. No new patients to be accepted after twenty-four hours of continuous duty

5. One day in seven free from patient care and educational obligations, averaged over four weeks, inclusive of call

6. In-house call no more than once every three nights, averaged over four weeks

If you do the math, you'll see these restrictions would still allow a resident to work a five-day week of sixteen-hour days, coming in at 6:00 in the morning and leaving the hospital at 10:00 at night. Assuming the resident requires a conservative thirty minutes in the morning and evening for changing clothes, showering, and commuting to and from work, that expands each workday to a seventeen-hour day, leaving only seven hours for sleep. Now tack on some quality improvement project the resident has to complete by the end of the month and the never-ending studying required to keep up with his rotations and to prepare for board exams, and we're left with maybe six hours for sleep. That's not leaving a single minute during the workweek for conversation with a spouse, relaxing with some mindless TV, or exercise. And yet this is still perfectly legal under the *new* work hour restrictions.

In reality, most residents work six-day workweeks, with the eighty hours averaged over those days, with some sort of overnight call thrown in every few days. Most of the days off are used for studying and catching up on sleep—maybe a trip to the gym or an outing with family. Copious time to pursue elaborate hobbies is just not there.

Another caveat about the work hour restrictions is home call, a sneaky type of call that sounds good—it has the word "home" in it—but can actually be a nightmare. In my surgery months during intern year, I had to be at the hospital by 6:00 a.m., was usually there until at least 6:00 p.m., and every few days had home-call duty. This meant my pager was fair game for any and all pages from nurses caring for every surgical patient. I got calls all through the night to place orders for fluids, sleep aids, EKGs, and so on. I occasionally had to go in to the emergency department for consults. And accounting for all of this time is tricky, as it doesn't count toward the eighty hours unless you are physically in the hospital.

Residency programs have made great strides in using residents' time more efficiently and intelligently. When today's retired physicians went to residency, residents often worked ninety to a hundred hours per week or more. They were lucky to get a few days off per month, with no guarantees of *any* time off. Hospitals used residents as cheap labor in the most extreme forms, making them perform all blood draws and start IVs in lieu of hiring phlebotomists or additional nurses. I know some hospitals still use residents this way. Even during my own residency, I frequently had to push back against the attitude that it was easiest to "just call the resident" to start an IV that looked difficult or to transport a patient after hours.

One of my attendings said things were so bad during her residency that she more than once worked in the OR as an anesthesiology resident well over thirty consecutive hours. Once she was so tired that she placed an auxiliary blood pressure cuff on her arm and set the time to every five minutes just so it would wake her up if she nodded off.

Things generally aren't *that* bad nowadays. But they're not great either. Aside from the cushiest specialties and specific programs, you should assume that for the majority of your residency, you will be working in the hospital around sixty-five to seventy-five hours per week, maybe getting one full weekend off per month plus one Saturday and one Sunday free each month—a total of four weekend days. With few exceptions, most residency programs don't bend over backward to give you much *more* than the required ACGME work hour restrictions.

Residency life is typically a bit better for specialties with few emergencies, such as dermatology, psychiatry, and physical medicine and rehabilitation. But it's typically worse for specialties with a heavy component of inpatient care or anything to do with surgery. Two of the largest fields, internal medicine and pediatrics, fall into this category.

Even surgical fields that seem like they may be lifestyle-friendly, such as plastic surgery, are almost always very time-consuming. Most folks think of plastic surgeons as doing nothing but breast augmentations and nose jobs—not so. Plastic surgery residents typically share all sorts of soft tissue trauma call and are constantly getting called into the OR in the middle of the night to assist with reattaching a finger or to operate on someone who burned his face off during a fireworks show.

Sometimes residency gets easier the more senior a resident gets. But this isn't always the case. Newer modifications to the ACGME work hour restrictions have actually placed even tighter restrictions on interns, meaning senior residents have to pick up the slack. And as residents progress through residency, they gain more useful medical knowledge and skill.

Imagine two anesthesiology residents still in the hospital at 5:30 p.m.: (1) a first-year resident on his first OR rotation and (2) a senior resident with years of experience working with critically ill patients. An eighty-four-year-old with a ruptured abdominal aortic aneurysm rolls through the trauma bay. Which resident do you think is going to be asked to stay late to help with the emergent case? In reality, probably both, since the junior resident can learn a lot from such a case. But the senior resident certainly isn't going home any time soon.

Both these residents may have planned on dinner with their families. But it doesn't matter. And that is perhaps one of the most annoying things about residency—certainly for significant others, if not for the residents themselves. As a resident, you have virtually no control over your time. You have a few precious days of vacation and protected time during which you cannot be called into the hospital. But at many resident programs, you will constantly be asked—or "strongly suggested"—to stay late or come in early for some educational gem of an experience.

Not that there isn't some truth to this. If I were one of those two residents, I would surely have stayed to participate. With better monitoring and endovascular repairs of abdominal aortic aneurysms, we hardly ever see emergent aortic ruptures anymore. Experience managing the complicated hemodynamics of such a patient would be a welcomed opportunity.

Unfortunately, there's almost always some great educational experience or reason to stay. And a resident can't really tell the attending, "Nah, that's okay. I'm pretty good on that, thanks." It's typically an offer you can't refuse.

MAKE EVERY MINUTE COUNT

My residency advice is to take advantage of every last free minute available to you; it is by far the most precious thing in your life. If you have a few hours during the day without clinical obligations and have tried studying but can't find the motivation or concentration, then put the books away and use your time some other way. There is absolutely no reason to waste time with a book on your lap if you're not retaining any information.

Get outside and enjoy the sun, spend time with friends, share a meal and conversation with your significant other, read a story to your kids, have an adult beverage if you're not on call. Hobbies are enormously beneficial. Residents in my class partook in a range of activities including boating, skeet shooting, running, beer brewing, ping-pong tournaments, poker, and flying stunt kites on the shores of Lake Michigan. (That last one was one of mine.)

STRESS MANAGEMENT

Speaking of unhealthy diversions, every year dozens of physician residents in the United States are treated for drug or alcohol abuse. Unfortunately, several residents die each year from such abuse. Likely due to a combination of high stress and easy access to narcotics, residents in my own specialty of anesthesiology are particularly susceptible to opiate abuse. Two residents in five years fell victim to this in my own residency program, and one died of an overdose a few months after my graduation.

Nearly all residency programs offer free or inexpensive mental health counseling services. If you struggle with the stress, isolation, and fatigue that often accompany residency or know someone who does, it is imperative to seek help. I have known too many residents who have attempted to cope with these pressures by abusing alcohol, taking out frustrations on their loved ones, or stoically bottling everything inside.

The good news is that residency goes by quickly and is over before you know it. The bad news is, the rest of your life goes by quickly during those years, too. And you'll never get it back, no matter how hard you try.

ANOTHER DOC'S SHOES: IT'S ALL ABOUT "ME TIME"

"Make time for yourself." This advice is dispensed to med students and residents ad nauseam. Since most medical trainees are young adults, its importance goes beyond simple stress release. Their identities are still being formed, and it's easy to lose oneself in the ultra-marathon of becoming a doctor. (What can I say? I'm a child psychiatrist.) Most folks recognize the value of this advice but laugh and say, "Yeah right, who has the time?" To this end, I offer some practical advice. You need to find two types of activities that interest you: those you can do in short increments while at the hospital or in class, and more time-consuming activities that can only be done outside of work.

"At work" activities can ideally be done quietly, with minimal equipment, and in brief spurts of five to thirty minutes. Examples include creative writing, puzzles, video games, nonscience reading, meditation, and drawing. "Outside work" activities take a little more time and should be scheduled events, preferably with other people (social pressure forces you to commit your time). Examples include team sports, book clubs, playing in a band, art class, yoga, and exercise classes. Finally, for all you über-competitive types: remember that "me time" activities should be about having fun and recharging—not overcoming personal challenges or being the best. Save that mojo for medicine!

JASON BURNS, M.D.
MEDICAL SCHOOL: University of Iowa, Iowa City
RESIDENCY AND FELLOWSHIP: Medical College of Wisconsin, Milwaukee

27.
JOLLY GOOD FELLOWS

"Yes, Ma'am; May I Have Another?"

Once a physician has completed residency in his or her chosen specialty, that individual can now happily go out and practice medicine as an attending physician—a bona fide doctor. But there's yet one more element of medical training we haven't discussed: a *fellowship*. A physician can pursue this optional training after completing residency. Fellowships can last anywhere from a single year to four years; during that time you are called a fellow.

CLINICAL AND RESEARCH FELLOWSHIPS

Most fellowships are *clinical fellowships*, similar to residency, though usually with better hours, more autonomy, less menial work, and often with research and teaching duties. On the medical totem pole, fellows rank somewhere between residents and attending physicians. I once saw an internet cartoon that said it can sometimes be difficult to distinguish attendings and fellows in a hospital environment, but you can differentiate from their cars in the physician parking lot. Indeed, most fellows are on the same pay scale as residents, making just slightly more money each additional year of training.

Clinical fellowships typically lead to subspecialization, as the physician acquires the additional procedural skills and knowledge needed to practice in a more highly specialized area of medicine than his or her original residency training. Such fellowships sometimes require additional board certification and exams at the end.

Research fellowships usually run for one or two years, are not clinically oriented, do not lead to clinical subspecialization, and center on completion of one or more research projects. Most research fellows work closely with a research-focused attending physician at an academic medical center, often serving as a primary assistant for his or her projects.

Many research fellows are international medical graduates attempting to gain experience in the American medical system, either to bring back to their native country or to gain acceptance to an American residency program. The latter approach would be to ultimately practice medicine in the United States. Unlike clinical fellowships, which are usually governed by the ACGME as are residency programs, research fellowships are most often independently run by academic medical centers and not bound by the same rules and regulations as ACGME-accredited clinical fellowships.

WHY DO A FELLOWSHIP?

Why would anybody pursue *optional* years of additional medical training? After all, the typical physician has already spent about eight years *after* college in various forms of medical training before even getting to the point of starting a fellowship. Why commit even more years of one's life? Why forgo potentially hundreds of thousands of dollars of income? Well, for one or more of four main reasons: money, job satisfaction, academic interests, and the job market.

Money

In general, *specialists* (any physician who specializes in a non–primary care field) make more money than primary care physicians (a.k.a. *generalists*). In some cases, the differences can be quite profound, with the highest-paid specialists earning several times what a generalist physician earns. Unless one completes residency training in a specialized field, such as anesthesiology or orthopedic surgery, you must complete a fellowship to become a specialist.

An example of using a fellowship to specialize is the case of an internal medicine resident (a generalist) who's completed a three-year fellowship in gastroenterology. That physician is now considered a gastroenterologist instead of a general internist. On average, a gastroenterologist makes several times the income of a primary care internist. Some might complete multiple fellowships to pursue additional subspecialization, like an interventional cardiologist who acquires the necessary skills by completing first a fellowship in cardiology, then a second in interventional cardiology. That's four years of medical school, three years of internal medicine residency, three years of cardiology fellowship, and one final year of interventional cardiology fellowship.

Job Satisfaction

Imagine an internal medicine resident who falls in love with the kidneys and renal physiology. She finds more enjoyment during all of her nephrology elective rotations than in any of her time spent on the general medicine floors or in the critical care units, cardiology wards, or pulmonary clinics. She knows she would be happiest specializing in the care of patients with renal disease. As such, she decides to pursue the required additional two years of fellowship training to become a nephrologist. Her primary incentive is likely not money—nephrologists usually earn salaries fairly similar to those of general internists—but rather enjoyment of the work and lifestyle. Of course, many physicians are passionate about—and complete fellowships in—specialties that also boost their incomes. The decision to pursue a fellowship is almost always multifactorial.

Academic Interests

Physicians also pursue fellowship training to become more competitive for positions in academic medicine. While it is certainly possible to work at an academic medical center as a generalist, academic superstars more often have a specialist niche, becoming an expert on a specific topic in their specialty. Indeed, most fellowship programs require fellows to complete a variety of research and teaching projects, so parlaying fellowship training into an academic medical career is a somewhat natural progression for those so inclined.

Job Market

Some residents decide to pursue fellowship training during a sluggish job market. If a physician finishing residency in a given field is entirely committed to staying in a specific geographic region, and he cannot find any suitable jobs in that area, then spending a year or two earning some money, adding a specialization to his CV, and potentially continuing forbearance of his loans beats working at a coffee shop.

A PERSONAL DECISION

I struggled with whether to do a fellowship, so I empathize with physicians who pursue additional training. You've already committed many years and countless hours of your life to your career as a physician. When you finish residency, you don't want to settle for just any available job. I decided during my anesthesiology residency that I would enjoy my career more if I could focus on patients undergoing cardiac surgery and procedures. After completing my residency I pursued an additional year of training in a cardiothoracic anesthesiology fellowship. Some positions reward cardiac-trained anesthesiologists with additional monetary compensation, but that's not always the case. I was motivated by improved job satisfaction, increased job opportunities, and a potential niche in academic medicine. Furthermore, larger hospitals in metropolitan areas increasingly require fellowship training to perform specialized duties. I didn't want to risk being unable to practice cardiac anesthesia in the future due to lack of training.

If you have any inkling that you want to pursue a fellowship, I recommend you do it immediately after residency. I know people who practiced as attending physicians for several years, then later decided to go back and complete a fellowship. But I can tell you from personal experience, it's best to have a rising income and standard of living. The pay cut you'll likely take, going from an attending to a fellow, can be brutal! Once you get out of training, grow your family, get a house, and generally accumulate required monthly expenditures, that pay cut may not be palatable or possible without dramatically affecting you and your family.

ACGME ACCREDITATION

Another fellowship consideration is ACGME accreditation. This is more of an issue with some specialties than others. Some fellowships are ACGME accredited; others are not. While I would never recommend attending a non-ACGME accredited *residency* program, it is a bit different when it comes to fellowships. Some fellowships are not ACGME accredited simply because the ACGME does not offer accreditation in that fellowship program. A rare fellowship type, offered in only a handful of programs, may not have garnered ACGME attention; the subject material may be so new the ACGME has not had time to catch up.

In these cases, attending a non-ACGME fellowship may not be a horrible thing; it might even benefit you. ACGME-accredited fellowship programs are hamstrung by a variety of rules and regulations. Some, such as work hour restrictions, can work in your favor; others, such as restrictions on moonlighting and simultaneously serving as fellow and attending, can work against you. Fellows in non-ACGME-accredited programs often work part-time as an attending physician at their institution, potentially doubling their income during fellowship. Fellows in ACGME-accredited programs can't do this.

Consider whether attending a non-ACGME-accredited fellowship program will affect your ability to become board certified in your subspecialty. For example, a few years ago the National Board of

Echocardiographers (NBE) restricted board certification in advanced perioperative transesophageal echocardiography *only* to graduates of ACGME-accredited cardiothoracic anesthesiology fellowships. You can still take and pass the exam if you complete a nonaccredited fellowship, but you cannot become board certified. This might matter, depending on where you want to work and what you want to do with your board certification. These types of issues will vary dramatically between specialties. Perform your due diligence and make sure you know what you are getting into before signing on any dotted lines.

DAILY LIFE OF A FELLOW

Life during fellowship is generally *much* better than during residency — in terms of hours, lifestyle, and autonomy. At most programs, you are no longer considered first and foremost a workhorse for the hospital. Not that you aren't still a cog in the machine of academic medicine, but compared to residency, you usually have much more time to devote to studying, research interests, and teaching residents and students.

Again, you are a notch higher on the medical education totem pole, just under the level of attending physician. That makes life at the hospital a lot better. At least now there's only one tier of people who can make you do their work and stop you at any time to ask you esoteric medical trivia. Meanwhile, you now have all students, interns, and residents at your disposal to do your grunt work.

Do your homework when comparing fellowship programs. While most treat you appropriately at a fellow level, some are notorious for abusing fellows, essentially treating them as additional residents. This varies by specialty; ask around within your field to identify the problematic programs.

Finally, you need to be wary of becoming too subspecialized, unless that is what you are looking for. For example, let's assume you are completing a general surgery residency and desperately want to work in a rural area of central Pennsylvania. Pursuing a fellowship in transplant surgery probably isn't going to be consistent with your career goals, unless there happens to be a major transplant center in rural central Pennsylvania. Being overqualified for your desired work location or practice setting is a very real concern when considering how deeply to subspecialize.

All in all, I greatly enjoyed my fellowship experience. Having an additional year after residency to focus on a specific patient population—in my case very sick and critically ill cardiac patients—helped strengthen my foundation as a general anesthesiologist. I appreciated gaining a deeper understanding of cardiac surgery, echocardiography, and various tools of the trade, such as the cardiopulmonary bypass machine, extracorporeal membrane oxygenation, and ventricular assist devices. It was also nice being able to stay in an academic environment while completing my written and oral anesthesiology boards, as well as during preparation for and completion of my perioperative echocardiography boards.

Fellowship isn't for everyone. Your choice whether to complete one will likely be shaped heavily by your specialty, career goals, ideal practice environment, desired geographic practice area, the current job market in your area of interest, and your degree of interest in academic medicine. If you have any significant inclination that you want to complete a fellowship, I urge you to pursue it right away after residency—*not* years down the line, when a massive pay cut and decreased status on the medical totem pole may complicate the picture.

PART IV

MEDICAL PRACTICE

28.

GET A JOB

Light at the End of the Tunnel

Sometime during the first few months of your final year in residency or fellowship (if you choose to do one), you will start looking for a "real job" as an attending physician. This can be frightening for some, especially those who have never actually had a normal job and have been in some form of education or medical training since preschool. Indeed, some find ways to delay the plunge into the working world, deciding to pursue additional fellowships, start over with a new specialty, or possibly matriculate in another degree program, such as an M.B.A. or master's in public health.

The world of medicine provides many opportunities for the "professional student." Sometimes these academic ventures can be financially rewarding. For example, I've known some physicians who initially worked in relatively low-paying specialties such as family practice or pediatrics, but decided to go back to residency to work in more highly paid specialties. Others get business degrees and make scads of money in private industry or with some entrepreneurial efforts. But for the most part, the endless education and underpaid training programs sought by professional students serve little purpose but to expand knowledge and enable their addictions.

Thankfully, the mere process of earning a medical degree and completing a single residency (and possibly fellowship) is usually more than enough to cure even the worst professional students. Once you finally are done adding letters after your name and board certifications to your credentials, it's time to dust off your old CV, brush up on your interviewing skills, and start looking for a job!

PREPARING FOR THE JOB SEARCH

Searching for your first job as a physician is much less formal and procedural than applying to medical school, residency, or fellowship. There are no standardized application forms or computerized matching systems. In fact, many of the best jobs never get published anywhere, but are advertised only by word of mouth.

When, where, and how you find your first medical job varies depending on your specialty, whether you are interested in an academic position or private practice, and in which part of the country and type of place you want to work. The application process generally starts toward the beginning of your last year of training, whether residency or fellowship. Accordingly, it's good to prepare a few months before that.

These preparations include getting your CV up to date; securing any letters of recommendation or references you may need; and locating and organizing all of your medical licenses, board certifications, diplomas, immunization records, and any other documents you may need to apply for jobs and become credentialed at a new hospital. Recall my advice to get into the habit, early on, of scanning into digital form every official document you receive from any of your prior colleges, medical training sites, state licensing agencies, and even your malpractice insurance documents. You will be amazed at how many times in your career you will repeatedly need to submit these documents to various interested parties.

ACADEMICS VERSUS PRIVATE PRACTICE

Many people will tell you the first step in the job search is to choose between academics or private (also called "community") practice. There are certainly differences in the two types of practice, but I don't agree that this sharp distinction must be made for all people. The boundaries between academic and private practice have become increasingly blurred in recent decades. In my personal experience, I considered academic positions within my geographic scope alongside private positions, evaluating all factors including geography, lifestyle, finances, patient and case mix, and practice environment.

Still, some people do need to settle this up front, as it may have a greater impact on the job hunt. For example, if you are a graduate from an MD-PhD program or are certain you want medical research to be a large component of your career, then academic medicine is clearly better for you. But if you hated working with medical students and junior residents during your medical training and cannot imagine spending another minute in your practice answering trainees' questions or watching a medical student struggle through some procedure, you should stay away from anything academic.

For most folks, the reality is somewhere in between, and I encourage you to consider all options with as open a mind as possible. For example, some community hospitals have arrangements with nearby academic medical centers, allowing some students and residents to rotate through their facilities for additional clinical exposure, perhaps specifically for a glimpse of the differences between academic and private practice styles. You could find a private practice position with many of a community hospital's benefits, plus the opportunity to become an adjunct faculty member of the academic center and occasionally work with students and residents.

Similarly, academic medical centers are increasingly under pressure to finance their research and educational missions through clinical productivity. There is a trend at many teaching hospitals to hire some physicians mainly to perform clinical work efficiently, allowing them some flexibility from the normal requirements that academic physicians research, publish, and teach.

The other typical differences between academic and private practice positions concern the types of patients and medical cases you will encounter, as well as employment and payment logistics. Though some private hospitals are busy tertiary care centers with very complicated patients, you will likely deal with more complicated patients and more uncommon surgeries and procedures (including transplants and high-acuity trauma) at academic centers. Some people may find the bread-and-butter nature of work at community hospitals less satisfying professionally.

Academic physicians are usually employees of the academic medical center. Physicians at community hospitals or clinics are more likely to have some ownership of their practice (hence the term *private practice*), but they are also increasingly employed by hospitals or large practice groups. Community physicians generally earn more than their academic counterparts, but the degree of difference varies by specialty, geographic location, and practice environment. Finally, academic centers often tie some portion of income to nonclinical functions including research productivity, teaching projects, and administration duties, whereas private practice physicians' incomes are largely, if not entirely, based on clinical productivity.

GEOGRAPHIC DECISIONS

The next big decision is where you want to work. What part of the country? Rural or metropolitan environment? This decision will depend on personal factors, such as proximity to family and friends, desire for exploring a new part of the country, or climate preference. However, some practical concerns also come into play.

In general, there is a perversely inverse relationship between physician pay and cost of living. This is in contrast to most professional careers, which typically feature higher salaries in cities like New York, Chicago, and Los Angeles, which is in part why those places are more expensive to live in. Because physicians are needed everywhere but more are found in some areas while other areas struggle to recruit them, physician pay varies from region to region. Most reports place the highest salaries in the Northwest, Central, Great Lakes, and Southeast regions, and the lowest salaries in the more expensive Mid-Atlantic, Northeast, and West Coast regions.

There are similar pay differences between metropolitan and rural areas. If your clinical practice is highly specialized or you want to perform only unusual procedures and see patients with esoteric diseases (the "zebras"), you're pretty much stuck with large hospitals in cities—or perhaps a handful of major research hospitals in rural "hospital towns." But if you're open to the idea of practicing in a rural setting, you will likely find a greater number of available jobs, higher starting salaries, bigger signing bonuses, more offers of loan forgiveness, more benefits, and more vacation. Of course, some people intrinsically desire a rural practice, so the financial benefits are a bonus.

POUNDING THE PAVEMENT

Once you've decided on a geographic area and whether you are open to academic jobs, community positions, or both, it's a matter of getting your CV out there and talking to as many people as possible to locate job openings. Look online and in medical journals and magazines. Some specialties have specific resources that are well known among people in the field. But again, some of the best jobs are never posted and are spread only by word of mouth. Groups typically fill these positions quickly.

To find out about these jobs, talk to colleagues in your specialty who are already out in the working world—either faculty at your training site or recently graduated residents or fellows. People who have just finished training and found jobs within the last year or two are more likely to know which groups are hiring. Someone like that in your geographic area of interest can be invaluable. If you are interested in academic positions, senior faculty in your department will often have connections across the country and can help put you in touch with the right people.

There are several medical recruiting firms who will undoubtedly tap you by phone or email at some point in your training. Recruiters have a larger role in some specialties compared to others. I didn't use them, but some classmates found their first jobs from recruiting firms with reasonable success. Hospitals or private groups pay recruiters for their efforts, so more of the recruiter jobs are likely to be hard to fill. This may be due to geographic location or factors like high job turnover and low job satisfaction. Recruiters are paid when they successfully recruit physicians to jobs, so always do your own research and never rely entirely on anything a recruiter says about a specific job.

If you are interested in military positions or jobs in the VA system, contact hiring personnel at the department of interest. Each military branch has medical recruiters who are more than happy to help. You can also search for military and VA positions at www.usajobs.gov; enter your specialty name (for example, "psychiatrist") and geographic area of interest. I know many people who are very happy with jobs in the military and VA systems, but working for the federal government comes with its own considerations. Talk to people already in the system before you sign up.

Medical career fairs are another resource. These are held regularly in cities around the country, and you will likely get emails or phone calls about such events during your residency or fellowship. If not, try a quick internet search for an upcoming event near you. These are very helpful for certain types of physicians, such as hospitalists, emergency physicians, and family practice doctors. I found them less helpful for anesthesiologists, but your mileage may vary. In general, the specialties more commonly employed directly by hospitals or health care organizations in your geographic area will be most represented at career fairs. If nothing else, typically there's a decent spread of hors d'oeuvres.

A less frequently used option is cold calling. Most graduating residents and fellows aren't terribly comfortable with this, but it can sometimes yield good results. One resident called the main operator at each hospital in the city he wanted to work in, asking to speak with the person responsible for hiring anesthesiologists. He usually got transferred to the on-call anesthesiologist for the day. Sometimes he learned the group wasn't hiring, but occasionally he got the name and number of the hiring contact. From there, he could get some leads to groups that were hiring, a few requests for him to send his CV, and ultimately an interview and a job.

Finally, don't forget about your own training facility. Many graduating residents and fellows find their first job at the academic medical center where they trained. Some find it a perfect fit and end their careers as bona fide academic physicians. For others, it's a way to get their feet wet as an attending in a familiar environment, prior to moving to a local private practice or perhaps going to a different city altogether.

The benefits to this option include starting your career working in a familiar setting with (hopefully) friendly faces. But you risk never entirely shedding the perception of you as a more junior partner — always the "former resident." I suggest exploring your other employment options before communicating with your own department. Otherwise, you might have to fend off daily inquiries about your response to a job offer while you are still figuring out the other options.

Though most potential employers want your CV submitted electronically by email or through a website, it can't hurt to print at least a dozen copies of your CV on some fancy resume paper so you have a printed copy available if you need it. Bring these along to career fairs and other events. And of course, always dress professionally. Business casual attire is probably sufficient for recruiting events and career fairs, but a suit is best when meeting with physicians from a specific group you are interested in. Remember that you are always being judged when meeting with potential employers, whether it is an actual interview or not.

TIMELINES

Nothing about getting your first real job as a physician is as regimented and rigid as the process of applying to medical school, residency, or fellowship. For example, I know one resident who had signed a contract with an anesthesiology group before he even started residency! He was from a small community in the Upper Midwest with a perpetual shortage of specialists, and once he had been accepted to a residency program, the chief of the local group guaranteed him a job upon completion of residency if he came back to his hometown.

In general you will start sending your CV to groups and hospitals in the fall of your final year of training and start hearing back in the late fall or early winter. If you're lucky, some responses will be positive! Many employers will want to chat with you on the phone first, or perhaps have you come out to the hospital or clinic to meet members of the group informally. Again, always dress professionally at such meetings. You will never be criticized for being too formally dressed, but underestimating the dress code could be a deal-breaker.

If all goes well, you will receive some interview offers. These typically start in the late fall or winter, but remember that private groups and community hospitals and clinics aren't operating on the typical academic medicine calendar. They may not know their staffing needs until later in the year, so timing is sometimes difficult when searching for your first job. Your dream job may not be available when you receive the bulk of your job offers. And by the time it is available, you may have already signed on with someone else. That's just the way it works sometimes for your first job. A surprisingly large percentage of physicians leave their first full-time position in less than three years.

INTERVIEWS

Interviews are usually as much an attempt to sell the job to you as they are an inquiry into whether you are a suitable employee or partner. You will typically have some flexibility in choosing your interview dates, mostly centered around whether the key decision makers in the group will be available to meet you. One of the tricky parts of the whole process is getting time off from residency or fellowship to travel to and attend interviews—something made even more difficult if you're looking to get your first job far away from your training institution.

The typical interview lasts one day, though there is often an informal dinner offered the night before or (more commonly) the evening of the interview. Hospitals and private practice groups will often invite significant others to these dinners, and they are a good way to meet some of your potential colleagues in a less formal setting. Potential employers are just as interested in how well you will fit with the group personally as they are about your clinical skills. If you've made it to this point, they will assume you are a knowledgeable and competent clinician.

Many groups will offer to pay for your travel and hotel expenses during the interview, and dinners are typically hosted at nice restaurants. I know that after years of abuse in residency, it can be easy to feel guilty for receiving such largesse. But take it in stride and just appreciate groups that do offer such gestures. You are a very highly educated and trained individual interviewing for a very well paid position with great responsibilities and expected professionalism. You will sometimes be interviewing with a small group, such that you will be only the third or fourth person in a small partnership. Your potential employers have the same degree of interest in attracting a professional individual who will be a good fit for their organization as you have in being hired by a fair, professional group.

Just as with interviews for residency and fellowship positions, job interviews are generally stress-free. To my knowledge, there are never any clinical questions asked or attempts to humiliate or trick interviewees. If you experience this sort of thing, I would be highly cautious about accepting a job from such a group. As I said, it's as much a process of the group getting to know you as it is giving you a good sense of the job, practice environment, patient mix, and financial details.

Regarding financial details, you shouldn't hesitate to ask for specific information on the day of your interview. If you've made it this far, the group is seriously considering hiring you or taking you on as a future partner. You have every right to ask for specific answers to questions regarding pay structure, salary, benefits, malpractice coverage, vacation, and becoming a partner if applicable. Don't settle for generalities at this point. Groups shouldn't have any reason to hide specifics from you, as these are all important things for you to know when comparing job offers.

ANOTHER DOC'S SHOES: HITTING THE INTERVIEW TRAIL

Unless you plan to do a fellowship, your final year of residency means it's finally time to start looking for your first real job as a doctor! If you're like me, you never had a "real job" prior to entering med school. I did some odd jobs in high school, served tables during college, and worked in a research lab during med school. I never worked in any corporate jobs where I had to go to interviews dressed in a pantsuit with a leather notepad clutched under my arm. So I had no idea what to expect once I started interviewing for doctor jobs.

In reality, interviewing for jobs as a physician was much more laid back than any of my other medical interviews up to that point, including those for med school and residency. Sure, I dressed up and was always professional. But there were no grilling questions or intimidation games. The interviews were mostly casual conversation with current docs in the group, tours of the clinics, and a few questions to get to know me better. I did notice some outliers: if you interview with government hospitals or clinics, including the VA system, you can expect a lot more paperwork and bureaucracy, which I guess isn't surprising. But once you get past the initial forms and interviews with random HR types, it's pretty much the same as interviewing with smaller, private groups. Good luck!

"JENNIFER," M.D.
MEDICAL SCHOOL: The Ohio State University, Columbus
RESIDENCY: University of Wisconsin, Madison

An increasing number of physicians are being employed directly by hospitals, insurance companies, or some mixture of the two. Nonetheless, many physician-owned private practice groups do still exist. When navigating the job search, it is important to understand some differences in the financial logistics between these two practice models. It is also important to ask as many questions as needed on the interview day to fully understand how each group runs its practice. I can't say it enough: something is wrong if a group is secretive or evasive with its answers to your questions.

EMPLOYEE JOBS

The employment model is familiar to most young physicians, as most all residents and fellows are employees. It's not terribly different as an employed attending physician, but of course there are many more variables. Most employed physicians are paid by some combination of a guaranteed salary and productivity-based pay. The proportions may change with time. Sometimes new physicians just starting in a new practice are given a higher guaranteed salary, with the income becoming more dependent on productivity with time.

As an employee, there is typically no possibility of ownership in a practice, so there generally isn't any "buy-in" as there is with partnership-track groups. But some employers will have a vesting period, such that employees receive only a percentage of the total compensation amount each year, such as 80 percent the first year and 90 percent the second. Number of vacation weeks may also similarly increase throughout your employment.

Benefits and Malpractice Insurance

One advantage of being an employee is that the employer covers virtually all expenses related to clinical practice. This usually includes malpractice insurance, dictation and electronic medical record expenses, medical licensing and professional society fees, and continuing medical education expenses, and often some contribution to disability, health insurance, and retirement funds. In a true private practice model, most of these expenses are the individual partners' responsibility.

As a potential employee you should consider some important details about these benefits, particularly when it comes to malpractice insurance. A full discussion of malpractice insurance and its nuances is beyond the scope of this book, but I'll hit the high points. There are two types of malpractice insurance: occurrence and claims-made. Occurrence malpractice policies protect the insured against any claims related to actions performed while the policy is in place, regardless of when the claim is made. In contrast, claims-made policies protect the insured only against claims made while the policy is in place. To extend coverage beyond the life of the policy, "tail coverage" should be purchased.

It is important to know which type of malpractice insurance your employer offers. Claims-made policies are more common than occurrence policies; if they offer a claims-made policy, ask whether tail coverage is also included in the employment package. Some employers will pay for tail coverage, but only if you fulfill certain duties, such as remaining employed for a minimum period or giving adequate notice before leaving the job. Your potential employer should be transparent and honest about these details.

Noncompete Clauses and Contract Termination

You should also understand the noncompete clause found in many employers' contracts, which places practice restrictions on an employee after termination of the contract. For example, a hospital employer may dictate that a physician employee cannot solicit any new patients within ten miles of the hospital for up to two years after termination. Some noncompete clauses are very restrictive and effectively prevent an employee from seeking new employment in entire metropolitan areas for some period after leaving a hospital. Others may simply state that a departing employee cannot directly compete for any current hospital patients.

The enforceability of noncompete clauses is a perennial subject of debate among physicians. I've known physicians who have had difficulties finding a new job in their desired geographic area because of noncompete clauses. But I've also heard and read comments from lawyers stating that noncompete clauses are difficult to enforce in court. But if a group or hospital sends a threatening legal letter to a competing group that is considering hiring a physician with a noncompete clause, that new group will usually skip over that employee just to avoid the legal hassle, regardless of its legitimacy. So it's in your best interest to sign a contract *without* a noncompete clause, or at least one that does not severely restrict your ability to find new work and solicit new patients in the event of contract termination.

Finally, you should understand whether the contract your employer is offering you is limited to a set number of years, whether there's a renewal option, and under what conditions it can be terminated. Most employers will hire you with some sort of vesting or probationary period, with the expectation that if there are no unexpected problems during your initial years of employment, the contract will be renewed. Otherwise, you should know up front if your employment is by design limited to one or two years—to cover a long-term but temporary absence of another employee, for example.

PRIVATE PRACTICE JOBS

When interviewing with physician-owned private practice groups, most of these same issues still apply. But there are some differences. First and foremost, you need to understand whether the job you are interviewing for is partnership track. Most private groups initially hire new physicians as employees, which they may call associates or some other name. Either way, it means you're not a partner right off the bat—and thus are not eligible to share in the group's profits as the partners are. You also are unlikely to be given voting rights within the group. The question to ask is whether the position is expected to result in partnership, or if you are being hired only for a limited period of time, forever as an employee of the group's partners.

Partnership Track

If you are indeed interviewing for a partnership-track position, then you need to figure out the details. Most partnerships expect associates to work a set number of years before offering them a position as partner. This typically ranges from one to five years, depending on the geographic area, specialty, and type of group. Associates are usually required to pay some percentage of their gross income each year to the group partners as a buy-in to become partner. For example, a group may have a three-year partnership track, requiring associates to pay the group 50 percent of their income the first year, 35 percent the second year, and 15 percent the third. After three years, the group votes on whether to extend a partnership offer, assuming the associate has performed to expectations.

Benefits, Vacation, and Other Details

Partners in physician-owned groups must provide their own malpractice insurance, health insurance, retirement contributions, and all other expenses. Partners in some groups arrange group policies to take advantage of group rates. Some partnerships also hire administrators or an outside firm to manage this. Others allow partners to handle all affairs on their own. As a new physician interviewing with such a group, you need to understand what sort of arrangement the partners have for themselves and, more important in the short term, what benefits and malpractice coverage, if any, are provided to nonpartner associates. This can dramatically change the overall effective compensation package, and must be considered when comparing job offers.

Vacation is sometimes handled a bit differently in physician-owned groups; have this explained during the interview. You will likely have a set number of vacation weeks as an associate, with greater flexibility as a partner. Once a partner, you might have a set number of guaranteed weeks of vacation, with the option to gain additional time off simply by forgoing payment for those days. Some groups guarantee no vacation time to partners, but instead simply pay them only for their individual billable amounts or days worked.

All of the other points discussed with employee-model practices also apply to physician-owned partnerships. This includes different types of malpractice coverage, inclusion of tail coverage, noncompete clauses, and possible reasons for termination. Most groups will willingly volunteer all of these details to you on the day of the interview, or at least give you documentation that covers this. If a group is unwilling or unable to answer these questions, be concerned. Either they did not ensure that an appropriate person was present on the day of your interview, or they aren't being up front for a reason.

Beyond all the financial details, it's also important to understand the day-to-day logistics of the group. This may be more challenging for a new physician with no prior experience as a practicing doctor. The specific questions you should ask will vary depending on specialty. In general, you should leave your interview with a good understanding of which facilities you will be working at, your normal working hours, which types of patients you will be seeing, which types of procedures you will be performing (if any), whether you will be working with mid-level providers, residents, or medical students, a rough idea of your call schedule, and how you are compensated for call duties.

Clearly, job interviews include lots of information gathering. You meet your potential partners; they try to learn more about you as a person and explain all that information in just a few hours. You will probably go on a tour of the hospital or clinic. Bring a pen and notepad to take notes if you feel so inclined. Just be yourself and soak in as much as you can. Most groups will have already distributed your CV to those who need it, so there's usually no need to bring another copy.

After you interview for a job, the usual pleasantries apply. A thank-you note is a good idea, but in my experience most folks prefer email over a fancy handwritten note. Physicians are busy, and a paper envelope is more likely to sit in some hospital mailbox for a few weeks, whereas your email has a pretty good chance of being seen right away.

YOUR FIRST JOB OFFER!

You might hear from someone a few days after your interview, or weeks may pass with no communications. Sometimes a response is delayed because the group is waiting until their next monthly meeting to discuss your potential employment. If you want a status update at any time, feel free to email your contact person and inquire. You're never going to lose a job that was otherwise yours because you asked about it. Occasionally, a group may want letters of recommendation, reference contact information, or even a second interview before making a decision.

Getting your first real job offer will be one of the best days of your medical career! It's up there with passing your board exams, graduating from med school, and finishing your last call shift of residency. You will typically have between a few weeks and a month to respond to an offer. Unfortunately, as great as that news can be, there might be another job you like better for which you are waiting for an interview or employment offer. This is a tough spot, and you can certainly contact the group you are waiting on to see if you can push their timeline a bit. Again, groups are just as motivated to find good physicians as you are to find your ideal job.

Contract Details

Once you do receive a job offer, the group should send you a copy of the contract for you to review. You will often be asked to sign and return a letter of intent for employment, with a signed contract expected at some later date. This gives you an opportunity to review the contract carefully—and time to have a trusted individual review the contract, specifically someone with experience reviewing medical contracts. There are attorneys who specialize in reviewing contracts, and it's not a bad idea to pay the money for this service. It can save you a lot of headaches and thousands of dollars in the future.

The main reason for this review is to make sure you understand exactly what it says. The reviewer should be able to explain to you in lay terms what you are signing. You should understand the answers to all the questions described earlier. If anything is unclear or does not seem congruent with what was described to you in the interview, contact the group for clarification.

Regarding potential for contract negotiation, you should have a good sense of where you fit in the supply-and-demand curve for your specific specialty and job market. If you are considering an offer to practice neurosurgery in the middle of Alaska at a hospital that has been looking for a neurosurgeon for five years, you probably have a lot of pull and can negotiate some points. For an offer to work as a hospitalist in a crowded, desirable market with several residency programs down the street, you might not have as much bargaining power.

Unless you have prior working experience, you probably won't have much luck modifying things like years to partner or buy-in amounts. The partners who already had to go through the buy-in process are often reluctant to budge on this point. You will likely do better negotiating more short-term things like a signing bonus (make sure you understand the tax ramifications), relocation expense coverage, or even base salary. It never hurts to ask, and a group that is truly interested in you is unlikely to rescind an offer just because you ask for a reasonable negotiating point. They may say no and keep the original offer, but that's probably the worst that can happen.

Once you're happy with a contract from a desired job, sign on the dotted line and drop it in the mailbox! You'll probably have a barrage of additional documents to sign over the next few weeks, covering things like hospital credentialing, background checks, malpractice coverage, and benefits. If you were promised a signing bonus, you should receive that in the mail within a few weeks of completing all the documents.

WHEN YOU CAN'T FIND A JOB

Unfortunately, each year there are graduating residents and fellows who have gone through roughly a decade of medical training and invested hundreds of thousands of dollars in their educations, but cannot find a full-time position in their specialty in their desired geographic area. It really does suck, and it's horrible that supply and demand of the medical job market doesn't always work out exactly as new graduates would like. But if you find yourself in this position, you have to come up with Plan B.

If you used government loans to help pay for your medical education, you should know that the minute you're done with residency or fellowship training, your forbearance period ends and loan payments are due. That can be a few thousand dollars a month if you're like most new graduates. So you have to find something to do that at least pays reasonably well. Toiling away a few months in an unpaid research position or volunteering at a hospital aren't really viable options anymore.

Lower Your Expectations

You have four main options available to you in this situation, assuming you need to start earning something in the ballpark of a physician's salary. First, you can admit you're just not going to get your dream job right out of training. This might mean you need to broaden your geographic area of interest to include neighboring cities, nearby states, or rural areas. I've known plenty of residents who settled on a job in a part of the country they never would have considered, only to discover they love their new home and now have no interest in leaving.

It could also mean settling on a job in your general field but maybe not exactly the practice environment or subspecialty work you ultimately want. For example, if you did a fellowship in interventional cardiology but cannot find work in this field in your city of choice, you could settle for a job practicing general cardiology, perhaps with the understanding that you will start working in the cath lab doing interventional work once a position is available. You just need to make sure your contract is flexible enough that when you find your ideal job you can leave your current position with relatively short notice without any unexpected penalties.

Locums Tenens

Your second option is to temporarily pay the bills by performing *locums tenens* work. You're probably wondering, "What the heck is *locums tenens*?" Roughly translated from Latin, it means "to hold a place." Like everything in the medical profession, we have to use a fancy Latin phrase to express the everyday concept of working part-time. Really, that's all it is: part-time work. Locums work is frequently advertised online and in print journals, and there are recruiters and physician employment agencies who specialize in connecting groups looking for part-time physicians with like-minded doctors.

With a locums arrangement, you go through the usual process of securing hospital credentials, proving medical licensure in the state, and agreeing to a background check. The hospital or private group will then contact you on a weekly, biweekly, or monthly basis to give you some possible dates you can work at that location. You usually may choose which of these dates you want to work. Most locums work pays quite well, and it usually involves no after-hours or weekend duties. Of course, benefits and retirement plans are seldom included, but malpractice insurance is sometimes covered. For most physicians, the biggest downside of locums work is the lack of consistency. The work pays well when you get it, but there is no guarantee of how many days you will be offered work each month.

Work Outside Your Specialty

A third option is to use your medical training to work in jobs that are open to physicians from all specialties, such as an urgent care center or even some emergency rooms. You may be able to find full-time or part-time work in such practice locations that will at least pay the bills and give you some clinical experiences while you search for a more ideal practice.

Back to School

Finally, your fourth option is a classic solution in the world of medical education: pursue more medical training! There's almost always another year-long fellowship opportunity out there you can sign up for. You can add a toxicology fellowship to your emergency medicine residency. You can do an additional research fellowship year to follow almost any residency or prior fellowship. You can add an advanced ERCP fellowship to your gastroenterology fellowship. There are countless opportunities to become a professional student once you have your medical degree.

As bad as it can seem not having your perfect job lined up immediately after finishing medical training, rest assured that it's generally a short-lived predicament. Assuming you don't have any major skeletons in your closet that were responsible for your bad luck on the job hunt, you'll likely find something that meets your needs within a few months. Remember that community practices don't revolve around the academic medicine calendar. It's possible that a group with no interest in hiring in July or August will suddenly have a retirement or unexpected departure of a partner later in the year. You just need to keep your ear to the ground and have some patience.

One last thing: A *very* small percentage of you will finish residency or fellowship training and pursue a more entrepreneurial path by starting your own private practice. While increasingly uncommon, there are some brave new doctors who do this every year, and my hat's off to them. I'd love to discuss this mode of practice in more detail, but frankly, it's so uncommon for new graduates nowadays and varies so much from case to case, I didn't think I could do it justice. So if you fall into this increasingly small group of physicians, best of luck following the road less traveled!

29.
DOCTOR BEWARE

Scams, Shams, and Shady Groups

It's unfortunate I even have to write this chapter. But I can't write a book like this without warning future and current doctors-in-training of this reality. You will find private practice groups in every specialty that are run by physicians whose primary goals seem to be milking every last bit of profit out of their specialty and patients, working new associates and junior physicians as much as possible for their financial gain, and selling out their group to some deep-pocketed buyer the first chance they get.

It really is a shame, considering that the medical profession is being attacked on so many fronts by outside parties. We have government leaders who don't understand anything about health care or medical economics, third-party payers with their own priorities that aren't always in line with physicians or patients, and celebrities and media charlatans feeding the public with pseudoscience and medical nonsense that wastes precious time in clinic and at its worst costs innocent lives. The last thing we need are members of our own profession—other physicians—harming the profession with their greed, pulling up the ladder after they make their graceful exit.

As I stressed in the previous chapter, an honest and fair practice will be completely up front about everything. There should be no vague answers about how patients are distributed to new associates or junior partners. There should be no generalities regarding partnership buy-ins, expected incomes, vacation distribution, or call schedules. If your interviewer can't answer one of your questions, he or she should be able to get you in touch with someone who does or get you the answer in a timely fashion.

If you think a group isn't being completely transparent with you during the interview process and contract discussions, you need to investigate further. I'm not saying the group is necessarily bad. But you should at the very least seek out private conversations with some other newly hired associates or junior partners in the group, and ask them how things are going so far. It's unlikely they have much to gain by lying to you, so I would trust their responses.

PARTNERSHIP TRACK TO NOWHERE

Thankfully, shady groups are not the norm. But you must be aware of the small percentage of private groups out there that are run by a small number of "super-partners" at the top of the pyramid—often the remaining founding partners of the group. These groups recruit heavily each academic year, luring new graduates with promises of high pay, better schedules, and eventually full partnership. Sadly, many of these promises are never met—particularly the promise of partnership. Instead of contributing buy-in for partnership, you will simply line the pockets of your group's existing partners with a large portion of your billings. Then your buy-in period will near an end, and your group will regretfully inform you that due to economic conditions or some other vague reason, they unfortunately cannot offer you a partnership position at this time.

On your interview days, be wary of groups with a large number of young, recently graduated associates, especially if all the partners are mid- or late-career. This doesn't necessarily mean the group is manipulating new graduates, but it should be a warning sign. Try to engage in a candid conversation with some of the junior associates. If the group is not in the same city as your training institution, talk to some practicing physicians in your specialty from the group's city. Reputations develop quickly when private practice groups consistently engage in this type of behavior. Do your due diligence; you should be able to steer clear of bad groups.

You should also be aware of the growing trend of physicians being employed directly by hospital groups or by regional or national staffing firms. If a group you are looking at is already a hospital-employed group, then there's not much to worry about. You are interviewing with the hospital and will simply become another employee of the hospital if offered a job. However, be wary of joining a private practice and committing to multiple years of a partnership-track, buy-in process if there is a good chance that the group is currently in the process of being purchased or absorbed by the hospital. You can imagine how you could end up giving your partners large sums of money during your buy-in period, only to have the private practice group dissolve just before you are offered a partnership. In some cases, the existing partners get a buy-out package from the hospital. Needless to say, if you are not yet a partner, there's little chance of your getting any of this money. So not only have you given large portions of your billings to your partners—who also benefited from the group converting to a hospital-employee model—but you also are never going to actually become a partner and benefit from the direct profit sharing promised to you.

THREAT OF A HOSTILE TAKEOVER

Large national and regional staffing firms are increasingly infiltrating physician markets in all specialties. This presents another risk for new residency grads just trying to find a job and start paying off loans. To understand this risk, you need to appreciate how most private practice groups interact with hospitals and clinics. There is usually a contract between the private group and the hospital to provide exclusive services in a given specialty. The hospital keeps all hospital charges; the group keeps all physician billings. Some contracts also include subsidies paid to the group from the hospital to compensate the group for nonbillable services, such as in-house call coverage or administrative tasks. The private group distributes its billings among its partners and nonpartner associates however it sees fit.

The tricky part is that these contracts are written for a set amount of time, often between two and five years. Every few years, the partners of the group and the hospital must renegotiate the contract. In decades past, this was basically a steak dinner and a few drinks, followed by a handshake. Nowadays, it's quite a different story.

In the era of increasing medical cost containment, every year hospitals are demanding more services for less money. Competing private groups in the same market have historically played nice in this environment, rarely attempting to undercut local competitors during contract renegotiations. This makes sense, since in a local market with only a few hospitals or a handful of clinics, most physicians in a given specialty likely know each other and remain fairly collegial.

However, the same civility doesn't exist with national and regional medical staffing groups. Many of these were founded by a small cadre of physicians but are now large, publicly traded corporations. Shareholder returns and profits are valued much more than long-term stability for the employed physicians or hospitals. The deep pockets of these groups have allowed them to approach hospital administrators during contract renegotiation cycles with promises of greater staffing numbers and more services with fewer or no hospital subsidies.

Hospital administrators need to contain costs, like everyone else, so these promises of more for less often are enough for hospitals to sever ties with private groups they have contracted with for decades. Sometimes the results are good; other times, the staffing turnover and disruptive changes in patient care cause problems for years after the deal is made.

For the individual physician, this creates yet more professional instability. As in the example of the private group absorbed by the hospital before you reach partnership, if contract renegotiations come up prior to your partnership date, you could be two years into your three-year buy-in period when you suddenly learn that your hospital won't renew the contract with your group, instead opting for an outside staffing firm willing to provide the services more cheaply. Your buy-in is wasted, and your private group no longer exists.

It isn't easy for a new graduate to predict any of these events. It would be wonderful if all private practice groups were completely forthcoming to interviewees about the length of time remaining in their contracts, whether they have discussed any possibility of selling their group to the hospital, or whether there is any strong concern of competition from a national or regional staffing firm. An honest and fair group will tell you these things, especially if you ask. It's up to you as the interviewing candidate to do just that.

Again, seek out practicing physicians in your specialty working in the market you are interviewing in. Rumors are sometimes just rumors, but there's reason for concern if you consistently hear that a group is bad to work for, a hospital contract is likely up for grabs, or a private group wants to sell out. On your interview day, don't hesitate to ask a group such questions. If you are a good, hard-working candidate, an honest group will never pass you up because you ask these questions.

ALTERNATIVE STRATEGY: WORKING FOR THE MAN

Concern about starting work at a private group that won't exist when it comes time for you to become a partner is one thing. What about starting right away as an employee of a hospital or a national staffing firm?

If you are reading this as a current pre-med, medical student, or even young resident, chances are good that you *will* end up working as an employee for your first physician job. That is the trend, and I don't foresee any reversal in the near future. The trend is advancing at different rates depending on specialty and geographic location, but advancing nonetheless.

Hospital Employment

I wrote quite a bit about the ins and outs of being a hospital employee in chapter 28, "Get a Job." Full disclosure: I am currently such an employee.

I have been happy with things so far. Certainly, there are issues at my hospital as with any job. But overall, I feel my specialty group is reasonably represented at the hospital level, our compensation is fair, and our benefits are generous. One advantage of employee status is the lack of cyclical insecurity each time contract renegotiations come up. It's also nice to have an employer take care of most administrative affairs including licensing fees, malpractice, and benefits. Finally, there is the benefit of being an employed member of the institution, as opposed to being an external group constantly having to interact with the hospital from the outside.

Downsides to hospital employment exist, as well. In this model, physicians are no longer independent practitioners paid for medical services by their patients (usually by way of insurance companies or Medicare). Instead, physicians' paychecks are written by large corporations, which are frequently complex unions of regional insurance companies and nonprofit hospital networks. Power lies with the people writing the checks, in this case hospital administrators—who themselves often report to insurance executives. All of this results in a loss of physician autonomy and the potential intrusion of corporate interests into the physician-patient relationship. At a more personal, pragmatic level, employed physicians do not have the same freedoms as their private practice colleagues in managing staffing, finances, reimbursement, facility and equipment purchases, or negotiations with hospitals and clinics.

Staffing Firm Employment

I can't address the specifics of working for a national or regional staffing firm from personal experience; in my specialty and my geographic area, such groups are not very prevalent. That isn't the case in all parts of the country. And other specialties in my area are frequently staffed by national firms.

I personally would rather either (1) be a partner in a physician-owned group and have the benefits of true ownership and control, or (2) willingly relinquish that control and ownership for the security and organizational integration of being directly employed by the care network in which I practice. I worry that as an employee of a national or regional staffing firm, I have neither the ownership and control that comes from private practice nor the organizational integration and security that comes with hospital employment.

Indeed, hospital groups can still dump their contracts with national staffing groups just as quickly as they can with a small local private practice group. But your mileage may vary. And in any event, the business of medicine will march on to its own drummer just as it always has. Hospitals will employ increasing numbers of physicians. National and regional staffing firms will continue fighting local groups for contracts and buying up independent practices. The old-school model of a small group of single-specialty physicians owning a clinic and managing all aspects of their practice will become increasingly rare. The really old-school model of a solo practitioner will become even rarer.

Maybe that's not all bad. Nearly all surveys in the last decade demonstrate that most young physicians leaving residency and fellowship have minimal interest in owning their own practices. Most prefer the simplicity of being an employee, focusing on clinical practice rather than managing the business of a clinic or hospital group. This isn't surprising, as increasing government and insurance regulations have made the business of running a clinic increasingly onerous.

I wish I could say that you don't have to worry about these types of things after working so hard to get into medical school, devoting countless hours of your life to your education for so many years, and incurring a quarter-million dollars or more of debt. Alas, I would be lying if I said you're inevitably going to stroll out of residency or fellowship and easily find the perfect job that will compensate you fairly if you work hard and practice what you learned in all your years of training. Just remember to look out for yourself, listen to those who have done it before you, and don't ignore your gut if you get a bad feeling about a potential employer or practice.

30.
SPECIALTY BOARDS

"It Costs *How* Much to Prove I Know Stuff?"

By this point, you've done well enough on the MCAT to get into med school, passed all four steps of the USMLE to get your medical license, and finally finished residency. You've easily spent thousands of hours studying for and taking all these exams. And you're about $5,000 poorer after all the exam fees and travel expenses. That doesn't include the cost of any study materials or review courses, which can easily rack up another grand or two in expenses.

Now it's time for your specialty boards!

That's right: there's one more set of gargantuan exams you have to take to prove that you learned enough about your specialty during residency to practice independently in your chosen field.

How much is that going to cost you? A lot, of course!

Internal medicine residencies always graduate the lion's share of residents each year, so let's first look at their board exam. According to the American Board of Internal Medicine, the 2017 fees to sit for the general internal medicine board exam are $1,365. If you do a fellowship and have to take a second exam for your subspecialty certification, that will cost you an additional amount: between $2,200 and $2,830 depending on the specialty.

In my specialty of anesthesiology, I had the privilege of taking both written *and* oral exams to become board certified. Per the American Board of Anesthesiology, the 2017 fees for the written exam are $1,550;

the oral exam costs $2,100. That doesn't include travel and hotel expenses, as the oral exam is held only in an office building near the ABA headquarters in Raleigh, North Carolina. All told, I'm sure it cost me somewhere around $4,000 to become board certified in anesthesiology. My subspecialty perioperative echocardiography certification was a steal at only $175!

HISTORY OF THE BOARDS

Though you will hear otherwise, board exams are actually *optional*. In decades past, becoming a *diplomate* (someone board certified in a professional specialty) in any field was considered a special distinction. It was optional for those practicing in a field to demonstrate their superior mastery of knowledge and clinical (for doctors) decision making.

As with many things in medicine, what was once optional is now essentially required.

Understand: No state has any law requiring physicians to be board certified in their fields in order to practice their specialties. In fact, a medical license alone is sufficient to legally practice any type of medicine you want!

Unfortunately, hospitals, clinics, and malpractice attorneys aren't so laissez-faire. If you were to hop right out of medical school without a residency under your belt and set up shop taking out appendixes, the first time anything went wrong you would have your pants sued off.

For many years, completion of residency alone was considered sufficient training to avoid such legal retribution. But board certification has increasingly become the expected standard. That's not to say there aren't thousands of physicians in the United States practicing their specialties without board certification. There most certainly are. But it's becoming less common, and recent graduates from residency are finding consequences to not being board certified within a few years of completing residency.

For example, many private practice groups explicitly state that they will not offer partnerships to associates if they have not become board certified by the end of the buy-in period. Similarly, many hospitals require board certification within a certain amount of time from initial employment to become a fully vested employee. Other practices will withhold a percentage of income if a physician is not board certified within a set period.

In short, if you're a new physician just starting your career, you must do everything in your power to become board certified in your field. If you've made it this far, you should be able to without any problem. You just need to put in the time to study and become familiar with the exam, its content, and the associated logistics. If an oral exam is required in your specialty, it's critical to reach out to some of your senior colleagues—ideally, actual oral board examiners—to ask them to help you with mock oral exams. I know, it sucks to intentionally torture yourself for practice, but you'll be happy you did when it comes time to take the actual exam.

DETAILS AND LOGISTICS

Board exams vary depending on the specialty, but there are many shared features. You are typically eligible to sit for your specialty's board exam sometime toward the end of your final year of residency, if not early in the first year out of residency. Many specialties then also require an oral exam, usually taken within a few months after passing your written board exam. Regardless of specialty, you'll fork out at least a few thousand dollars for all these exams.

Some advice regarding board exams: First, some employers will reimburse you for fees related to becoming board certified, partly because it's in their best interests to have board certified physicians on staff. Save all your receipts, even if you are still in residency or fellowship while paying for these exams. You never know; your future employer might help defray those costs.

Second, taking specialty boards is just like every other standardized medical exam you've taken by this point. Get familiar with the exam, its content and layout, and the timing of the exam. Find a review book that you like and study it. Ask people who have recently passed the exam which study materials are most reflective of the current exam.

Finally, make special preparations if your specialty requires an oral board exam for certification. If you're like most physicians, you haven't taken a lot of oral exams in your training. It's very different from slogging through the typical multiple-choice exam. Practicing by taking mock oral exams is key. If you know a physician in your field who is or has been an oral board examiner who can conduct these, even better. Chances are at least one former or current faculty member of your residency or fellowship program has been one. It's not fun being formally pimped by a colleague, but it's key to success on the real exam. You will learn the format, your weaknesses, and potential pitfalls to avoid.

You'll discover at some point there's controversy among physicians about the necessity of board exams, whether the whole thing is a big money-making racket for the specialty boards, and the injustices of some senior physicians being "grandfathered" out of the requirement of taking board exams. None of this really matters. It makes for interesting conversation, but in reality board certification is increasingly considered a requirement for fully independent practice in this country. If you're smart, you'll take your boards right out of residency while all the information is still fresh. Then you're done with it and can forget about it.

31.
STARTING YOUR FIRST *REAL* JOB

"Where's My Attending?"

Starting work as an attending physician is an indescribably wonderful experience. In my case, I completed my specialty and subspecialty board exams during fellowship, so I was completely free of all remaining vestiges of medical training when I started my current job. That sense of freedom of not having yet another massive exam looming ahead is something I hadn't felt in almost ten years. And it was extraordinary!

Unfortunately, the sense of relief and excitement that comes with finally being done with medical training is quickly tempered by the realization that for the first time ever, you are really and truly practicing medicine with *nobody* looking over your shoulder. The buck stops with *you* now!

NOBODY TO CALL

By this time, you have undoubtedly made many medical decisions and probably performed a fair amount of procedures in residency without direct attending supervision. There are those middle-of-the-night ICU orders, the after-hours central line placements, and the myriad pages from nurses every day of your residency that elicited quick responses ordering a bolus of fluids here or a dose of medication there—all without your attending physician checking in every step of the way.

But part of the process of medical training is giving you the knowledge and experience to know when things can go bad quickly and when you are working at the upper limits of your skill level. You are trusted throughout your residency and fellowship years to know when you need to call your attending for a second opinion or a second set of eyes to make sure you're doing everything right.

Once you're an attending physician, you suddenly realize how comforting it was to have that second opinion and second set of eyes just a quick phone call away. No longer can you ask the nurse to call your attending when you're having difficulty with a procedure or a patient is not responding to your treatments the way you expected. All eyes and ears are on you, and it's up to you to do what's right for your patients.

To be sure, if you've joined a good, collegial group of physicians, you won't be thrown to the wolves on day one. I have nothing but positive things to say about how helpful all of my partners were during my first few months as an attending anesthesiologist. Sometimes it was as simple as running my plan by a colleague to make sure it wasn't completely out of left field. Other times, it was a colleague coming in to provide a fresh set of hands on a challenging epidural placement or a difficult airway. Be wary if you interview with a group that gives you the impression that you will be entirely on your own with no help from your partners. That sort of attitude doesn't benefit anybody, least of all your patients.

LEARNING THE ROPES

The logistics of your first day at work will vary depending on your specialty and practice type. When I began as a hospital employee, I spent a few days in orientation activities. By contrast, most of my colleagues who started in physician-owned groups spent an hour or two touring the hospital and getting badge access, thereafter immediately starting work with patients. Either way, the process of learning the geography, names, and faces of a new hospital environment never changes. You've done it dozens of times in med school, residency, and possibly fellowship, and this is no different.

Chances are good nowadays that you'll have some sort of electronic medical record (EMR) system wherever you start working. If you haven't used it before, that will take some getting used to. Then you'll have to start learning names and faces of the many nurses, physicians, and mid-level providers you'll interact with. You're the new physician on the block, so everyone will know your name. But you will likely still be learning everyone else's names a month or two later.

ANOTHER DOC'S SHOES: A FRESH START

It has been said that starting a new job is one of the most stressful life events one can experience. Those people probably aren't doctors . . . Sure, moving to a new town, starting a new practice, and making new friends sounds stressful, but for doctors, the years of anticipation of "life after training" seem to help ease this transition. Not to mention the increased pay for (likely) shorter working hours and the freedom of practicing without an attending looking over your shoulder. Starting your first *real* job is gratifying.

It has also been said that learning never stops. This saying, unlike the first, most certainly applies to young doctors. I can say with certainty that I learned as much about myself and medicine in my first year of practice as I did in all my years of residency. For most, it is the first time out of a particular hospital system or "training gene pool"—a circumstance that demands flexibility and humility. Things as minor as IV needles or as major as hospital policies may be rather different from those learned during training, which requires adaptability and, again, humility. Thankfully, the medical trainee has spent years perfecting these very virtues, which, again, helps to ease the transition. Starting your first *real* job is edifying.

KYLE MORGAN, M.D.
MEDICAL SCHOOL: Ross University School of Medicine, Portsmouth, Dominica
RESIDENCY: Medical College of Wisconsin, Milwaukee
FELLOWSHIP: Children's Hospital of Wisconsin, Milwaukee

There's certainly a lot of pressure to make things go as smoothly as possible early on. My advice: Keep things simple, do what you feel is safe, and don't try to impress anyone by being a cowboy, taking on more than you can handle, or experimenting with unusual or new techniques. A disastrous medical error resulting in patient morbidity or mortality in the first year of your practice can be devastating. It can hurt your confidence, ruin your reputation, and bog you down early in your career with legal and administrative headaches—not to mention the emotional trauma and responsibility of causing harm to a patient.

As long and torturous as medical training can seem, I have been amazed at how well my training prepared me for independent practice. Most residency and fellowship programs are at teaching hospitals with high-acuity patients, including patients with nonexistent medical care, trauma patients, transplant recipients, and patients with rare and exotic diseases. You'll find that you've actually been exposed to almost everything you'll see in private practice at one time or another. So when it's just you and a nurse with a patient in the middle of the night, you'll somehow know what to do because you've done it many times before.

Of course, there will always be some diseases or procedural cases more common in your new practice than in your training. If you work in private practice and leave the world of academics, you might find that the supposedly simple bread-and-butter stuff is what you're least familiar with. But all of that can be learned on the job. You have to trust that your medical training up to this point gave you the skills to adapt to new clinical challenges and use your available resources to learn new techniques and treatments.

Again, never hesitate to ask your colleagues for help. Even if you don't know your new partners well, you can always call or email your old residency colleagues about any clinical problems you've encountered. They'll usually appreciate the question, as it's likely a situation they have encountered or will encounter themselves sometime in the future. And of course, many of your nurses and mid-level providers have been working with your new patient population much longer than you have. They may know some of the patients personally, and you can learn from their experiential wisdom. Use your resources to their fullest.

LOSING THE TRAINING WHEELS

The first few months will likely fly by. With each passing week, you'll know your way around the day-to-day logistics better. You will surely make some mistakes; some may humble you as a physician. You might even experience the death of a patient. You will learn from your mistakes and become a better physician because of them.

Before you know it, practicing medicine without someone looking over your shoulder will be second nature for you. You will anticipate problems sooner, work more efficiently, and improve your diagnostic and procedural skills every day. You will gradually develop your own style, pulling from everything you were taught in your training and from your new experiences as an attending.

Congratulations! You're finally a *real* doctor—*really*!

32.
YOUR FIRST ATTENDING PAYCHECK

"What Do I Do with *This*?"

What better way to follow a chapter about your first job as an attending physician than with a chapter about your first *paycheck* as an attending physician? Indeed, one of the biggest differences you will notice as an attending physician is the sudden increase in your income. The medical profession is most similar to pro sports and the entertainment industry (though on a much smaller scale) when it comes to dramatic changes in income occurring almost overnight.

Depending on your specialty and practice environment, you will see your annual income increase anywhere from three- to ten-fold in the first year of practice as an attending physician, compared to your final year of training.

So what do you do with the sudden influx of cash?

MORE INCOME, MORE EXPENSES

First of all, you should realize that in some physician-owned private practice settings, you may not see any substantial amount of money until a few months into your practice. In practices that pay you directly from your clinical billings, it can take a month or two before the money is actually collected from Medicare and insurance companies. Some groups will provide you some guaranteed income that you will receive right away, or they might allow you to borrow from the group's earnings against your expected earnings until you have an established income stream. Hospital employees may have a similar scenario, such that you might get paid your guaranteed salary right away but will not receive any productivity-derived pay until several months after you start your job.

In addition to the possibility of delayed payment, realize that if you are with a physician-owned group, you will be responsible for many expenses related to your clinical practice. This includes malpractice premiums, equipment expenses, licensing and credentialing fees, and your own health benefits. You may also be expected to contribute a significant portion of your income as a buy-in for your eventual partnership. Some groups take these expenses out before you get paid; others expect you to handle these payments on your own. It will all work out in the end, but you need to consider these things when estimating your initial monthly income. You can't simply take your promised annual income and divide by twelve.

Realize too that along with increased income come many increased expenses. If you have had government student loans in forbearance during medical training, the payments will become due as soon as you finish residency or fellowship—even if you have not yet earned any income from your new job. Average med school graduates these days have roughly $300,000 total debt by the time they start their first real job as a physician. This amounts to a few thousand dollars per month with most loan repayment plans.

INSURING YOUR INVESTMENT

If you haven't already done so, I highly recommend protecting your earning potential with good disability insurance. You have invested many years and hundreds of thousands of dollars in your medical education and training. Financially, that translates to nearly guaranteed employment with a significant earning potential. That's not a bad return on investment, but it can all be for naught if you suffer unexpected physical or mental injury or illness that prevents you from practicing in your specialty.

Many hospital employees and some associates of physician-owned groups will have some standard short- or long-term disability insurance included in their basic benefits package. But these are seldom sufficient to provide you with long-term security to maintain a similar standard of living if you can no longer practice in your specialty. Unless you are very comfortable navigating the world of insurance policies, find an insurance professional who works with physician clients and can help you fully protect your investment in yourself—someone you trust and feel comfortable working with. Ask your colleagues for referrals.

If you have a family, you will also want to secure appropriate levels of life insurance to protect your significant other and children. For most young, relatively healthy physicians, life insurance adequate to maintain a constant standard of living for your family in the unlikely event of your death is fairly affordable. This is especially important if you decide to reconsolidate government loans to acquire a lower interest rate, as most private debt passes on to your next of kin upon your death, unlike government loans, which are forgiven when the borrower dies.

Of course, as you add adequate disability and life insurance protection to your financial portfolio, that means more money out of pocket each month, as premiums can total several hundred dollars a month.

STUDENT LOANS AND DEBT RECONSOLIDATION

Many new physicians struggle with handling their student debt. Most who have finished residency within the last few years or will finish residency in the immediate future have government student loans with interest rates somewhere around 7 percent. That's not horrific, but it's not exactly good either.

Some of my colleagues who finished residency in the early 2000s were more fortunate. Many had government loans with interest rates as low as 2 percent. It's a no-brainer that you should pay those off as slowly as possible, as you're almost guaranteed to make greater returns by investing the money you otherwise would spend paying down your debt.

But what do you do with 7 percent? One option is to reconsolidate to obtain a lower interest rate. I described this process in greater detail in chapter 4; here I'll briefly recap. There are a handful of private lenders that specialize in providing loans to highly paid professionals with very good credit histories, including recently graduated physicians. You can search for some of these companies on the Internet and ask your colleagues for referrals.

These private lenders will ask for a lot of personal information, including bank statements, loan documents, usernames and passwords for all of your credit card online accounts, and documents from your new employer providing evidence of your guaranteed income or projected productivity-based income as a physician. Unless you have some financial skeletons in your closet, you will likely be approved for one of these loans. You can then reconsolidate your government loans, transferring them to the private lender for a lower interest rate, to be paid off within five to twenty years.

The benefit of reconsolidating your loans is that you can obtain a lower interest rate and potentially gain more control over how you pay off your loans and over what time period. Most private lenders also allow early repayment without penalty, so you can be more aggressive in paying down your debt if you find you have more discretionary income than you expected. The biggest drawback to these private loans is that you are now dealing with a private company, which can potentially be more difficult than dealing with a government lender. In particular, government lenders will forgive your remaining debt in the event of your death, whereas private lenders typically pass the debt down to your next of kin. Thus it's important, if you convert your loans to a private lender, to have adequate life insurance if you have a family.

If you do reconsolidate to a lower interest rate, you at least know you will now spend less money on interest over the life of your student loan. Next, consider how aggressively you want to pay off your loans. Some of my colleagues were very aggressive and put almost all their discretionary income into paying down their student loans. A few paid off all of their debt in less than two years—quite an accomplishment. Others choose a less aggressive strategy, chipping away over five, ten, or fifteen years.

Whichever method you choose, remember that if your lender allows early repayment without penalty, there really is no reason to commit yourself to an aggressive payment schedule—except for the possibility of obtaining a lower interest rate. For example, you can commit to paying $1,000 per month over fifteen years. You can have this amount automatically deducted from your checking account each month, which usually results in an even lower interest rate. But if you find you actually can afford to pay $3,000 per month toward your student loans, then you can just schedule an additional $2,000 payment each month without penalty. That way, if your expenses unexpectedly increase in future years, you can go back to the original $1,000 monthly payment.

LIFESTYLE CREEP AND UNCLE SAM

In addition to repayment of student debt and insurance premiums, your monthly expenditures will also increase due to the lifestyle creep that inevitably occurs as you adjust to your new income level. It's good to maintain your lifestyle as close to that of a resident as long as you can. After all, you've managed to live off that income for several years, so you should be able to do it for a bit longer. This allows you to more easily tuck away money for savings and repayment of your student loans.

But let's be honest. You've been working eighty-hour weeks for years, studying and taking dozens of exams, working in stressful situations making life-and-death decisions every day. You are now working as an attending physician, and all of your colleagues are going on nice vacations, purchasing nice cars, living in the best school districts, going to nice restaurants. It's inevitable that you're going to have *some* lifestyle creep no matter how hard you try to avoid it. If you keep this in mind, you'll be able to better plan your first year's finances.

Finally, there are taxes. Unless your spouse was in a highly paid profession while you were in residency and fellowship, you are about to pay more in taxes and various government contributions than you likely earned as gross income during your last year of training.

There's no way around it—taxes suck. And you're going to pay *lots* of taxes by the time you retire. Your effective tax rate depends on your specific financial situation: how much you earn, whether you are married, how many children you have, and many other factors. Your best bet is to plan conservatively the first year in practice until you go through your first tax season and get a good sense of how much of your income you actually keep. A good and trusted financial adviser can help optimize your tax burden, insure your income, and develop an overall financial plan.

RECEIVED WISDOM

To recap and add a few additional pearls of wisdom, here are the high points of my financial advice for new physicians:

1. Don't rush out and buy a sports car or a million-dollar home. It's fine to enjoy some things you've been putting off during your training now that your income has improved. But plan conservatively; wait and see how much you're actually keeping each month after taxes and expenses. Make sure you're not surprised on your first tax season as an attending. Once you have a consistent income, start making long-term plans and be more aggressive with your budget planning.

2. If you don't already have one, get a trustworthy financial adviser who is accustomed to working with physicians. He or she can help you avoid common pitfalls and develop a comprehensive financial plan.

3. If you haven't already done so, get good life and disability insurance. The disability insurance should support a comfortable lifestyle if you can no longer practice in your specialty. Be wary of policies that are very restrictive as to when they will pay out—or might even require you to practice outside of your specialty if you still can. Find a trusted insurance adviser—who may or may not be the same person as your general financial adviser.

4. Figure out what to do with your student loans. Pay them off aggressively if it gives you peace of mind. If you decide to pay them off more gradually, consider reconsolidating with a private lender to obtain a lower interest rate and reduce your overall interest expenses. If you do this and have a family, get adequate life insurance to cover the remaining debt in the unlikely event of your death.

5. Consider renting your home for the first year or two. I know, after years of putting things on hold for your medical training, it's tempting to rush out and purchase a home. And for many people, that may be the best decision. But don't feel like it's the only choice. I especially recommend this for people moving to a new city for their first attending position. I know several colleagues who thought they would love their first job, purchased a huge house in an unknown city, and within a year or two were looking for a new job and were stuck with an expensive house they couldn't easily sell.

6. Make sure you really like your new job and your new city, figure out exactly where you want to live, and save some money for a down payment. Just because your income is high, you might find that with your limited earning history and potentially large debt (in the form of student loans), you will have more difficulty securing a home loan than you expect. After the 2008 mortgage crisis, even young physicians with large salaries had trouble financing homes. If you can come to the table with a legitimate 20 percent down payment, it will be much easier.

7. Start saving now. Unless you had joint finances with a significant other who was working a normal job while you were in residency, you've probably saved very little money up to this point. You most likely earn enough now to cover all of your basic expenses, live a decent lifestyle, and still save a significant amount. At the very least, you should maximize your 401(k) contributions if this is available to you. More ambitiously, try to save 15 to 20 percent of your post-tax income off the top before spending anything. Depending on how conservatively you want to manage your money, "saving" can include paying down student

loans, saving for a home down payment, or saving for kids' college funds. But make sure you tuck away some significant portion of your income for something other than a fancy car, clothes, dining out, and vacations.

8. Before making any big purchases, notably a house, make sure you have a good handle on exactly what your monthly expenditures will be. Keep track of your expenses for the first year or so to have a good sense of how much money you are actually keeping at the end of each month. You can expect to pay a lot more in federal, state (if your state levies it), and property taxes than you're accustomed to. And expect some degree of "lifestyle creep" whether you plan for it or not.

9. Remember, when you first start working as an attending physician, you may not see all the income you expect right away. Associates of physician-owned groups who are paid largely from billed services may see nothing at all for a few months. Hospital employees may initially receive only guaranteed incomes, while a large percentage of their expected income will be paid as a productivity bonus later in the year.

10. Finally, remember that if you own your own medical practice or are a member of a physician-owned group, you will likely have some unexpected expenses related to your clinical practice. Malpractice insurance is a common one. Ask senior partners in your group if you have any questions.

33.
CONTINUING MEDICAL EDUCATION

"It Costs *How* Much to Prove I Still Know Stuff?"

You've been an attending physician for a year or so, and at this point you're really comfortable with your new position on the medical totem pole. It's been long enough since the trauma of med school and residency that you can think back fondly to your memories of graduating from medical school, passing your USMLE, getting your medical license, completing residency, and finally passing your board exams to become a board certified physician in your specialty.

Congratulations! Now you just have to maintain your continuing medical education. Oh, and let's not forget about Maintenance of Certification (MOC) for your specialty board!

"*What?!*" you exclaim. Oh, you thought you were done with all that? Of course not!

Medicine is no different from many other highly regulated professions in that you will spend the rest of your working life proving to your state licensing department that you still know enough and are up to date enough to continue practicing. This is known as *continuing medical education* (CME).

Don't worry. Your first year after completing residency or fellowship, you're good to go with CME. The fact that you just finished your medical training program is proof enough that you know what you're doing and are up to date on medical knowledge.

Beyond that, the specific details of how many CME credits you need and how often you need to report them vary from state to state. Check with partners in your group or consult the state licensing websites for information. Your state medical society is also a good resource. Finally, many hospitals employ an administrator responsible for maintaining physicians' CME and can help you determine how much you need to complete each year.

Thankfully, accumulating CME doesn't mean you have to publish a literature review or present a poster at a national meeting. There are many organized talks and workshops, often held in big cities or tropical locales, that allow you to attend a few lectures between ski runs or snorkeling and easily rack up some CME credits. There are also online lectures, review courses, professional society meetings, and other events that frequently count toward your CME credits.

DON'T LOSE TRACK

Keeping track of your CME credits is half the battle. That hospital administrator mentioned earlier can help. And as a bonus, many physician groups and hospitals will reimburse you (including travel and hotel expenses) for approved CME activities.

Yes, it sucks to have to keep track of these things. And I'm sure you would continue to read *JAMA* and *Annals of Surgery* religiously even though you're done with residency. But you have to do CME and keep track of your credits in order to keep your medical license. So just suck it up and do it.

But wait—there's more! Remember that board certification you got a while back? Over the last few decades, most specialty boards have established MOC requirements to ensure that their board certified physicians stay up to date not only with general medical knowledge but also in their specialty.

CME has been around for decades and has been mostly accepted by today's current batch of physicians. MOC, on the other hand, has recently garnered a lot of criticism from physicians across specialties.

Many argue that over the last decade, specialty boards have become increasingly onerous with their MOC requirements, are charging exorbitant fees, and have essentially turned MOC into profit-making ventures that physicians are forced to participate in by the de facto necessity of being board certified.

IT ALL ADDS UP

From the American Board of Internal Medicine (ABIM) website, the fee for a ten-year MOC subscription including the recertification exam required every ten years is $1,940, or $194 per year if paid annually. For my own specialty, the website quotes a price of $2,100 for every ten years of MOCA. Per the American Board of Surgery (ABS) website, the current fees for the ten-year MOC cycle for surgeons are $400 to apply for the exam and $1,100 to actually take the exam.

In general, most specialty boards seem to charge somewhere between $1,500 and $2,000 every ten years to maintain board certification. Traditionally, a recertification exam is required every ten years. In recent years, the ABIM and other boards have added more and more requirements to maintain certification, such as simulation sessions (typically held in one or two places in the country, requiring travel and lodging) and complicated schedules of learning modules and online assessments. Of course, the specialty societies that are often tightly connected to the specialty boards offer packages that help physicians easily fulfill their MOC requirements—for a cost.

Thus far, I've had only limited experiences with CME or MOC. I understand the argument that medicine advances so quickly that physicians' clinical knowledge and skills can become outdated and might benefit from an occasional refresher. But I also appreciate the increasingly common viewpoint of more experienced physicians that the entire process is becoming too complicated, expensive, and burdensome. It doesn't help that most specialty boards have "grandfathered" in their most senior diplomates (which always includes those in decision-making positions within the boards) as exempt from these MOC requirements.

In my own specialty, the ABA recently announced the release of what they called MOCA 2.0. This replaced the ten-year recertification exam with interactive learning tools that anesthesiologists must complete more regularly throughout each ten-year MOCA cycle. It also eliminated a required patient simulator experience—which would have required travel and lodging in Raleigh, North Carolina—instead making this optional. Diplomates still must complete CME credits and maintain good professional standing. Oh, and the $2,100 fee previously required every ten years for the recertification exam has been replaced with an annual $210 fee. I'm no mathematician, but . . .

In any event, along with CME, MOC is also probably here to stay. The good news is, specialty boards seem to be reversing the trend of increased requirements and costs, so it will probably be less onerous by the time most of you have to deal with it. But in the end, if you want to become and remain board certified, you'll do the same as you do with CME. Just suck it up and do it.

Are you starting to notice a trend when it comes to becoming—and remaining—a physician?

34.
WHEN THINGS GO WRONG

Guilt, Sleepless Nights, and Malpractice Attorneys

Physician paychecks come with physician responsibilities. Once you're out of the womb of medical education, the buck stops with you. With the exception of a handful of specialties, you will most likely work in a hospital or clinic setting with several members of a health care team. This includes mid-level providers such as physician assistants and nurse practitioners, nurses, technicians, pharmacists, and nursing assistants. These people are well trained in their areas of expertise and will surely voice concerns if they feel you are doing something that places patients at risk or is not standard of care.

In many cases, their concerns will be well founded. Perhaps you are working in a new facility and are not familiar with the equipment or formulary. Maybe the patient population at your new workplace is different from your training population. There will be times when patients require different clinical treatments from the ordinary approach. You may very well be doing something unfamiliar to other members of your care team with a specific therapeutic goal in mind.

We are increasingly working in an era of health care teams and cooperative medical decision making. However, ultimately you are the patient's physician. You are signing the prescriptions, performing the procedure, or managing the patient's overall care. If you feel an uncommon or riskier approach is best for a patient, that is for you and your patient to decide. As we also increasingly work in an era of informed consent, it is vital that your patients understand to the best of their abilities their clinical options, risks, and potential benefits.

Sometimes—hopefully most of the time—your clinical acumen will lead you down the right path and result in therapeutic success. However, there will be times when your decisions directly or indirectly result in patient harm or even death. Simple accidents or mishaps may also be to blame for patient morbidity or mortality. To err is human—and as much as patients and doctors like to think otherwise, physicians are human too.

THE WEIGHT OF RESPONSIBILITY

As a practicing physician, you are no longer able to shift the blame to your supervising attending. And while assistants and support staff are sometimes partly responsible for such errors, pointing fingers at them won't get you very far. When a patient experiences death, injury, or even lack of successful treatment, questions are first directed at the physician. The buck stops with you, and sometimes that pressure can feel like the weight of the world.

Practicing physicians deal with mistakes and failures in different ways. Some doctors overreact, vowing never to cause patient harm or death by the same mistake again. Their practice becomes increasingly conservative, sometimes to the point that aggressive but warranted treatment options are avoided to the detriment of patient care. Others attempt to shift blame elsewhere, to other physicians, ancillary staff, and sometimes to the patients themselves—blaming the failure of treatment on "unusual anatomy" or "faulty information provided by a consult." Again, doctors are only human, and subject to human defense mechanisms.

Perhaps most commonly, physicians internalize their true reactions when patient death or injury results from their actions. We are taught repeatedly throughout medical school and residency to separate our clinical experiences from our emotions and the humanity of our patients. We are encouraged to toe a fine line between empathizing with and relating to our patients and still treating them in a scientific and detached fashion. We are conditioned to appreciate our patients as biologic entities with physiologic and pathologic limitations that sometimes cannot be overcome.

Still, it is tough when a specific decision, action, or intervention made by us as physicians is responsible for harming or killing a patient. Sometimes we rationalize that the patient was very sick anyway and we only hastened an inevitable outcome. We might try to console ourselves by viewing the poor outcome as a learning experience that can improve our care and outcomes for future patients.

You never know how you will respond to mistakes and bad outcomes until you are in that position yourself. The specific reaction also depends on the nature of the mistake. Did you hasten the death of a terminally ill cancer patient by inducing a known side effect of a new, recently approved chemotherapy agent? Did you choose to wait just a few more minutes before taking a patient to the operating room for a cesarean section, only to discover that the baby was delivered too late and suffered anoxic brain injury? Or did you accidentally cut a major blood vessel during a complicated surgical procedure, causing the patient to lose massive amounts of blood and die on the operating room table?

Making mistakes as a physician can have profound consequences for patients, their families, and your coworkers. It can lead to feelings of guilt, defensive practice techniques, decreased confidence, questions of competency, and many sleepless nights. Some mistakes are so profound that they force physicians to stop performing specific procedures, treating certain types of patients, or practicing medicine altogether.

MEDICAL MALPRACTICE

While nothing is more serious and feared than injury or death of a patient, perhaps the only thing that comes close in its ability to keep physicians awake at night is the fear of a malpractice lawsuit. In August 2011, researchers from Harvard Medical School published a study in the *New England Journal of Medicine* that revealed some sobering statistics about medical malpractice. According to the study, one in fourteen

American doctors faces a malpractice suit each year. Moreover, almost every physician will face at least one malpractice suit during his or her career. Thankfully for physicians, analysis of over forty thousand physicians over a fourteen-year period showed that malpractice plaintiffs won their suits only 22 percent of the time.

Though medical schools are increasingly placing greater emphasis on the fiscal and legal aspects of medicine, doctors traditionally have received very little education about medical malpractice during their training. As such, most physicians lack even basic knowledge about what is required for a medical mistake or action to be considered malpractice. They are similarly ill prepared to intellectually or emotionally respond to malpractice suits when faced with them in their own careers.

In common law jurisdictions, the norm throughout most of the United States, a *tort* is a civil wrong that unfairly causes someone to suffer loss or harm, resulting in legal liability. Medical malpractice is a specific type of tort that relates to loss or harm secondary to medical treatment provided by a physician or other licensed medical professional.

As with all torts, medical malpractice plaintiffs must establish all five of the following elements of negligence to have any chance of succeeding in court:

1. A duty was owed. A legal duty exists whenever a hospital or health care provider undertakes care or treatment of a patient. Defendants named in malpractice suits must have actually been involved in the medical care of the plaintiff.

2. A duty was breached. The health care provider failed to conform to relevant standard of care. This is why expert medical witnesses are frequently called to testify in such trials, in order to clarify what is and is not within the standard of care given a specific clinical scenario.

3. The breach of duty caused an injury. The breach of duty must be a direct cause and the proximate cause of injury. A simple mistake that does not result in any injury to the patient is unlikely to result in a successful malpractice suit because there is no injury resulting from the breach of duty.

4. Deviation from the accepted standard. If enough medical witnesses can be found to convince a judge or jury that the physician's actions are within the normal standard of care expected from physicians within his or her specialty, given the clinical scenario, a successful medical malpractice suit is unlikely.

5. Damage. Some damage must result from the injury. This must be quantifiable into some monetary amount, but a number can always be produced, since it can include emotional damage, the latter part of "pain and suffering." More obvious damages include medical bills and lost wages due to injury.

When a patient tells a physician, "I'm going to sue you!" chances are the potential lawsuit will go nowhere. Though lawyers advertise on television all the time asking injured patients to give them a call, such attorneys know what constitutes a legitimate malpractice suit and what doesn't. The vast majority of potential plaintiffs who present their cases to malpractice attorneys are thanked for their time and sent on their way. There is no incentive for lawyers to spend time and money on a case that has no chance of even seeing a jury, much less winning in the court of law.

Of those cases that do have some legitimacy and meet the five elements of medical negligence, most never actually see a courtroom. There is usually a series of conversations between the prosecuting attorney and counsel from the physician's group, hospital, or malpractice insurance company. Depending on the facts of the case and potential damages of the proposed lawsuit, the case is often settled out of court.

A small percentage of malpractice suits actually see a courtroom, where the usual legal proceedings occur. Most of the time, multiple parties will be named as codefendants in the lawsuit—essentially any medical professional involved in the care of the patient who has assets personally or by way of malpractice insurance. This commonly includes nurses, physicians from different specialties such as the surgeon and anesthesiologist, licensed technicians, and mid-level providers. Though physicians are often the primary target due to their role as ultimate decision makers and their relatively deep pockets, any licensed professional involved in the incident is fair game.

Regardless of whether a malpractice suit actually makes it to court, the psychological and emotional toll on physicians can be intense. Thankfully, in the first year of my medical practice I have not yet been on the receiving end of a malpractice suit, so I cannot speak from personal experience. But physicians I have spoken to who have had to deal with the threat do not speak fondly of the process.

ANOTHER DOC'S SHOES: MIND YOUR OWN BUSINESS

Ethical dilemmas are common in medicine. A common ethics problem involves balancing the right to patient privacy with the safety of others who may be affected by that patient's medical condition. Every physician sees countless examples, even before the end of residency training. I once took care of a man dying of complications from AIDS. He had suspected he was infected for years, but he had forgone medical care and never had a formal test. Finally, he was forced to come to the hospital, received a positive HIV test, and was told that his wife and other sexual partners were required by law to be informed of his diagnosis.

He absolutely refused and insisted that his wife and family be told he was dying of lung cancer. He threatened to sue the hospital and everyone involved, and ultimately he threatened to kill himself if anybody found out about his diagnosis. Of course, we told his wife and reported his illness to the Centers for Disease Control, as required by law. He ended up spending some time in the psychiatric ward after his repeated suicide threats. He died of a severe AIDS-related infection a few weeks later.

"PATRICK," M.D.
MEDICAL SCHOOL: University of Florida, Gainesville
RESIDENCY: University of Wisconsin, Madison
FELLOWSHIP: Washington University, St. Louis, Missouri

Even if a lawsuit doesn't result in a trial, physicians feel a degree of personal insult and attack at the mere mention of a malpractice suit. There are inevitably countless meetings with hospital administrators, legal counsel, and insurance personnel. There are forms and potential probation of hospital privileges; rumors develop. The experience is typically described as time-consuming, degrading, insulting, exhausting, and scary. Unfortunately, statistics suggest every physician will encounter it at some point in his or her career.

When a patient experiences injury or death resulting from your actions as a physician, you should first contact legal counsel from your physician group, hospital, or other employer. Counsel may recommend that you contact someone from your malpractice insurance provider to give them your side of the story while things are still fresh in your mind. It is always in your best interest to maintain good relations with your patient (if still living) and his or her family. Be honest about what happened and be forthcoming with information. Malpractice defense attorneys tell me the worst thing you can possibly do as a physician is to alienate your patients in such situations and make them feel that you don't care about them, are trying to avoid them, or are trying to hide information from them. All else being equal, physicians who are well liked by their patients tend to be sued less.

According to the *New England Journal of Medicine* study mentioned earlier, the specific rates of malpractice suits varied greatly by specialty. On the high end, roughly 19 percent of neurosurgeons and cardiothoracic surgeons faced lawsuits each year compared to about 3 percent of pediatricians and psychiatrists. Mean indemnity payouts ranged from $520,923 for pediatricians to $117,832 for dermatologists.

I hope you will avoid a medical malpractice suit in your career or at least delay one until you have a few years of confidence-building experience under your belt. If you are still choosing your specialty, know that specialties involving high-risk procedures and high-risk patients come with a similarly greater risk of being sued for malpractice. Whatever type of medicine you will or do practice, remember that humans make mistakes, and all physicians are humans. As such, you need to accept that you will someday, somehow make a mistake that directly causes injury or death to one of your patients.

35.

OCCUPATIONAL HAZARD

Dealing with Death on a Daily Basis

Just as mistakes (and taxes) are inevitable, so is dealing with death as a physician. True, the frequency of daily interaction with death is greater for a forensic pathologist working in the morgue than for a dermatologist. But all physicians deal with death to some degree, and with a frequency much greater than in the average professional's career. If you are not already comfortable with the continuum of life and death, then you certainly will be by the end of your medical training.

Many medical students spend at least a few weeks learning gross anatomy by way of dissecting preserved human cadavers. This does a good job of desensitizing medical students to the concept of human death, as well as the act of cutting and manipulating human tissues for clinical purposes—in this case for the purpose of medical education.

But truth be told, cadavers bear only a partial resemblance to living humans. The skin is discolored, tough, and a bit shriveled from the formaldehyde preservation. The limbs are stiff from the rigor mortis. The bodies are motionless and clearly devoid of life from the very first time students see them.

CODE BLUE

It is often not until clinical rotations or even intern year that most physicians-in-training witness a patient dying before their eyes for the first time. Medical interns spend a great deal of time in hospitals overnight, frequently on medical ward teams that respond to medical codes. A code is an alert notifying in-hospital physicians and other staff that a patient is dying or in acute medical distress. When such an announcement is transmitted overhead or by pager system, everyone on the call team runs to the specified location, usually carrying some sort of backpack or case with rescue drugs, intubating equipment, and IV supplies.

I think my record for a single night on call was five legitimate codes. I use the word "legitimate" to distinguish from the "fake codes" that all medical students and residents come to know and love. These are code alarms dispersed throughout the hospital that are triggered by a janitor accidentally bumping against a button in the ICU or a sleepy patient pulling the wrong cord in a bathroom. They seem to always occur at 3:00 in the morning, directing everyone to the farthest reaches of the hospital, and are promptly canceled just as everyone arrives, short of breath, with adrenaline coursing through their veins. Believe it or not, most residents do get to the point where they can promptly go back to sleep after such an event.

On my overnight call with five codes, I felt like my medical team was bouncing back and forth from emergency room admissions to coding patients the entire night. The first was a woman having a persistent seizure. She had pulled out her only intravenous catheter, and the in-house anesthesiology resident finally secured an IV that enabled us to administer medication to break the seizure. The second code was an elderly gentleman found deceased in the bathroom by a nursing assistant. He was face-down in his own bloody vomit and was a bit chilly when we found him, meaning he had been dead more than a few minutes. He was labeled a "full code" (as opposed to a DNR or "do not resuscitate"), so we went through the motions for one round of cardiopulmonary resuscitation (CPR). But we all knew it was hopeless, so we quickly called the code and notified his family.

The other three patients were more typical codes, in that they had been alive in hospital wards or in the ICU and then, all of a sudden, were no longer alive. In normal circumstances, these people would be found the next morning motionless in bed, or perhaps their spouses would see them suddenly gasp for air and slouch over in their favorite chair. But in the hospital, critically ill patients are often monitored by cardiac telemetry or continuous pulse oximetry, so the moment of death is known immediately.

DETAILS OF DEATH

Everyone dies in some specific way. Laypeople will say a grandmother died of lung cancer or that a man died from complications related to an automobile accident. But things like lung cancer and automobile accidents don't *really* kill people—at least not directly. More precisely, they produce chains of events that ultimately lead to one specific thing that ends someone's life.

Sometimes electrolytes become so out of whack that the heart's conduction system stops functioning properly, resulting in a fatal arrhythmia that prevents the heart from effectively pumping blood, which starves all the body's tissues of oxygen, including the brain. This is what happens on television shows when paramedics or doctors yell things like, "He's in v-fib. Grab the paddles!" It's pointless to shock a heart that has no electrical activity and is doing absolutely nothing, as the point of the electric shock isn't to "jump-start" the heart but rather to interrupt the fatal arrhythmia, hoping that the heart will start back on its own in a normal rhythm more compatible with life. We did this with two of the remaining three patients during my busy call night, with successful conversion to a stable rhythm in one of the two cases. This sequence of events is played out with varying degrees of accuracy on television medical dramas.

Another possibility is that something occludes a patient's airway or prevents her from ventilating properly, which eventually results in reduced oxygen in the blood and, you guessed it, all of the body tissues becoming oxygen-starved. Eventually, the heart itself becomes oxygen-starved, which typically leads to slowing of the heart rate or a fatal arrhythmia, which hastens death. Thankfully, patients tend to lose consciousness pretty quickly in any of these processes due to lack of oxygen to the brain.

In the fifth coding patient of my busy night, a combination of cardiac and respiratory issues led to the patient's demise, which we couldn't reverse despite our best efforts. This patient had been recently diagnosed with cancer, which causes the body's blood thinning systems to get all out of whack and increases the risk of blood clots. The patient had been alive and well, watching late-night television, when her husband saw her suddenly grab her chest, report that she had trouble breathing, and moments later lose consciousness—again, due to lack of oxygen to the brain.

She had suffered the most fatal type of blood clot: a saddle pulmonary embolus. This is a big clot that usually forms in the deep veins of the legs and travels up the inferior vena cava, into the right atrium of the heart, through the tricuspid valve, into the right ventricle, and out into the pulmonary artery that delivers deoxygenated blood to the lungs. This blood normally flows through the lungs, where it becomes oxygenated and returns back to the left side of the heart, where it is forcefully delivered to the entire body to provide oxygen to all the tissues. A saddle embolus is a clot so big that it occludes most or all of the blood flow through both the left and right pulmonary arteries. It crams itself into the bifurcation of the main pulmonary artery like a saddle on a horse's back. This not only blocks blood flow through the lungs for proper oxygenation but also prevents sufficient blood flow through the heart at all. The result is lack of oxygen to the tissues, unconsciousness, usually arrhythmia, and death.

Ultimately, it's almost always something with the heart, the lungs, or the interface between those two organs that kills people. Yes, people can die of liver disease, kidney failure, strokes, cancer, or horrible infectious diseases. But in the end, it boils down to the A-B-C's: *a*irway, *b*reathing, *c*irculation. To stay alive, you need oxygen continuously delivered to your tissues—at least to the vital organs like the brain, heart, and lungs. Anything that impedes that process, such as obstruction of the airway, cessation of adequate ventilation, or disruption of circulation of blood (the human carrier of oxygen) results in death if allowed to persist for too long.

And that's how doctors all eventually come to view the continuum of life and death. Life is indeed mysterious, special—one might even say miraculous. But in a strictly physiologic sense, human life is the coordinated activity of all of our organs and tissues, made possible by production of energy, which requires nutrition in the long term and oxygen in the short term. Oxygen is obtained from the atmosphere through the airway and infused into the blood by juxtaposed capillaries and alveoli. Oxygen infused into the blood attaches to hemoglobin molecules, which are pumped by the heart to all the tissues in the body through the circulatory system. Oxygen is released to the tissues in exchange for the waste product of carbon dioxide, which is then pumped back to the right side of the heart and into the lungs to repeat the whole process.

If anything is left to stop any of these processes for too long, the entire house of cards comes crashing down, and what was alive is now dead. The brain is typically the limiting factor, as it can function without oxygen for only a brief time period. We can shock hearts to get rid of fatal arrhythmias, pump epinephrine into veins to increase blood pressure by squeezing the vessels and hopefully kick-start the heart into a normal rhythm. But every second the brain is not receiving oxygen, brain cells are dying. This is why the classic TV scene of doctors performing CPR on a patient for an hour and suddenly having that patient wake up and thank everyone for their efforts is patently ridiculous. The worst possible outcome is a resuscitated patient with a dead or severely injured brain, which does sometimes happen.

ANOTHER DOC'S SHOES: DON'T PULL THE PLUG

One thing I have learned working with many elderly and sick patients as a hospitalist is that the dying experience and expectations for the final days of life are extremely personal. Even after several years of training and practice, I'm still occasionally surprised. I once had a patient with end-stage liver disease who had become so sick and confused he required a breathing tube and ventilator in order to breathe. He did not have a living will in place, so his wife became his power of attorney and decision maker by default. She argued that he would not want to live in his current state and wanted us to withdraw care by taking him off the ventilator. His children disagreed, arguing for us to do everything possible. Given the circumstances, I thought the wife was being quite reasonable and figured he probably would not want to live dependent on a machine.

Much to the surprise of everyone on the medical care team, upon turning off the ventilator and removing the breathing tube, the patient became lucid for just a few minutes and mustered the energy to say nothing more than, "Put the tube back in. I want to live." Apparently his children knew his dying wishes better than his wife! Shortly thereafter, he wrote on a piece of paper that he wanted his oldest son to be his new medical decision maker.

"JAMES," M.D.
MEDICAL SCHOOL: Johns Hopkins University, Baltimore, Maryland
RESIDENCY: Virginia Mason, Seattle, Washington

HUMANITY OF DEATH

These scenarios of resuscitating patients, feeling ribs crack under your fingertips during chest compressions, seeing a patient's eyes roll back into his head before he takes his final breath, bringing patients back from life only to discover too much time passed without oxygen to the brain and care later needs to be withdrawn—these scenarios repeat over and over and over again during the many years of medical school, the intern year, and into residency. Depending on the specialty, some physicians take part in these frequently throughout their entire careers.

It certainly is possible to simultaneously be a physician and maintain a respect and appreciation for humanity and the uniqueness of human life. Many doctors maintain a deep religious faith, and some gain a great deal of comfort and professional guidance from their faith. But if you haven't already reached this point in your medical education, know that you will experience life and death in an entirely different way than you probably have thus far in your life.

Sooner or later, you will view the qualities of life and death—and the distinction between the two—differently than you once did. In some ways, the first half of becoming a physician is spent becoming comfortable with death and viewing human beings as physiologic machines. By contrast, the second half is remembering what it's like to not be comfortable with death and how everyone else views the miracle of life.

EPILOGUE

Many Grains of Salt

I wrote this book to provide a literary counterpoint to the countless books that answer the question: "How do I get into medical school?" This book is an honest portrayal of the many trials, tribulations, and triumphs I experienced in the past decade of my life, from the time I first decided to go to medical school until the present—just a year into practice at my first "real" job as an anesthesiologist at a busy community hospital. I hope this collection of thoughts, opinions, and experiences helps guide current doctors-in-training as they traverse the tumultuous waters of medical training. I also hope this book gives pre-med readers insight into what becoming a doctor is *really* all about.

If you are still wondering if becoming a physician is the right choice for you, I encourage you to speak to as many people in health care occupations as possible. Speaking to doctors is important, but you may be surprised to learn about other health care professions that interest you. Of course, you may ultimately decide medicine isn't your calling, and that's all right, too.

Please visit my website, www.medschooluncensored.com, and contact me with any questions about becoming a physician, attending medical school or residency, and life as a newly minted doctor. On my website, you will find some material that didn't make it into the book, including chapters on part-time opportunities, nonclinical careers for physicians, retirement, and special concerns for medical trainees with disabilities. You will also find detailed descriptions of alternative, non-physician careers in health care—including some jobs you've probably never heard of, such as perfusionist, ultrasonographer, and nurse anesthetist.

Finally, I wish you the best of luck in your endeavors. For those applying to medical school or who are currently in the process of medical education, I look forward to the day I can call you a physician colleague. If life takes you down a different path, then I hope you find success and happiness in your own way. Wherever life takes you, thank you for using your precious, limited time to read my book!

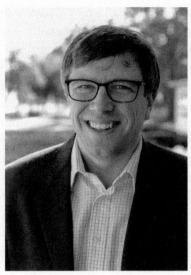

ABOUT THE AUTHOR

Dr. Richard Beddingfield is a practicing cardiothoracic anesthesiologist at a busy community hospital in Madison, Wisconsin. After a childhood spent in Florida and Georgia, he headed north for college, receiving a bachelor of business administration degree from the University of Michigan, Ann Arbor, in 2001. He spent a few years in a variety of white-collar roles, including cofounding a technology firm and managing tax accounts at a corporate insurance agency. Finally, he decided to go back to school to fulfill a dream first hatched during his senior year in college. He completed prerequisite coursework for medical school and took the MCAT in 2004.

Dr. Beddingfield earned his medical degree from the University of Minnesota in 2010, after which he moved to Milwaukee, Wisconsin, and in 2014 completed anesthesiology residency at the Medical College of Wisconsin. A lifelong student, he moved back to Minneapolis to pursue a fellowship in cardiothoracic anesthesiology at the University of Minnesota. Finally, he moved to Madison in August 2015 to start his first real job as a private practice anesthesiologist.

During his years of medical training, Dr. Beddingfield frequently taught and mentored other future physicians. As a chief resident, he introduced students and residents to the basics of anesthesia and the operating room. As a fellow, he instructed residents on cardiothoracic anesthesiology and echocardiography. He still has a passion for helping pre-meds, med students, and residents. *Med School Uncensored* is the product of that passion and the desire to help tomorrow's doctors maximize their educations and avoid common mistakes.

Dr. Beddingfield lives with his wife, Laura, and daughters, Lydia and Audrey. When he isn't at the hospital or writing books, he enjoys spending time with family, traveling, losing money at poker, and playing piano.

INDEX

prerequisite coursework
for, 21, 22
relationships and, 64–72, 189
starting, 60
undergraduate program
combined with, 20
See also admissions process;
allopathic medical
schools; Caribbean
medical schools;
curriculum; exams;
medical school students;
osteopathic medical
schools
medical school students
with children, 70–72
demographics of, 61–62
gunners, 89–90, 135–36
motivations of, 6–18, 27
sex lives of, 64–65, 67
social dynamics and, 63
Medical Scientist Training
Program (MSTP), 52–53
Medicare, 14, 39, 41, 231, 242
medicine
rotations, 122–30
as specialty category, 122
See also individual specialties
military
positions, 211
scholarships, 53–55
mistakes, 114, 127, 255–61
MOC (Maintenance of
Certification), 250–53
morning rounds, 122–25
MSTP (Medical Scientist
Training Program), 52–53

N

National Board of Medical
Examiners (NBME), 142
National Board of Osteopathic
Medical Examiners
(NBOME), 108
National Health Service Corps
(NHSC), 56
National Residency Match
Program (NRMP),
101, 149, 150, 153
NBME (National Board of
Medical Examiners), 142
NBOME (National Board of
Osteopathic Medical
Examiners), 108
nephrology, 78, 122
neurology, 103, 111
neurosurgery, 73, 78, 103,
149, 260
NHSC (National Health Service
Corps), 56
noncompete clauses, 217
NRMP (National Residency
Match Program),
101, 149, 150, 153

O

OB/GYN (obstetrics and
gynecology), 56, 103, 111,
112
occupational medicine, 122
ophthalmology, 76, 77, 102, 149
OR (operating room), 131,
133–37
orders, 125
orthopedic surgery, 73, 74–75,
102, 103, 122
OSCEs (objective,
structured clinical
examinations), 145

osteopathic (D.O.) medical
      schools
   allopathic vs., 41–43
   applications to, 34
   Caribbean vs., 47
   concept of, 40
   history of, 40–41
   residency and, 41–42
otolaryngology, 76, 103, 122, 151
out-of-state applicants, 28

P

partnership track, 218–19,
      227–28
part-time work, 223–24
pathology, 77, 103, 122
patients, standardized, 88–89,
      144, 145
PAYE (Pay As You Earn)
      repayment plans, 50
pediatrics, 56, 78, 103, 111, 122,
      194, 260
personal statement, 26–27
PhD. *See* MD-PhD
physical medicine and
      rehabilitation, 75, 77,
      103, 194
physicians
   as couples, 150–51, 188–90
   earning potential of,
      12–14, 199–200,
      209–10, 242
   ethical dilemmas and, 259
   financial advice for, 242–49
   health care teams and, 254
   malpractice and, 234, 256–61
   mistakes by, 255–61
   nonclinical careers for, 269
   reasons for becoming,
      6–18, 27
   as relatives and friends, 14–15
   respect and, 14

responsibility and,
      254, 255–56
   shortage of, 38–39
   specialist vs. generalist,
      199–200
   on television, 18, 64
   thinking like, 116–17
   See also attending physicians;
      job search
pimping, 115–16, 182
plastic surgery, 42, 78, 103, 194
post-graduate year (PGY), 163,
      167. *See also* residency
preliminary year, 163, 164, 167
"pre-med," meaning of, 22
primary care, 56, 111
private practice, 207–9, 218–20,
      225, 226–30
progress notes, 127–28
pseudoseizures, 126
PSLF (Public Service Loan
      Forgiveness)
      program, 51
psychiatry, 77, 103, 111, 122, 194,
      260
pulmonology, 122, 177

R

radiation oncology, 42, 78, 103
radiology, 77, 103, 111, 122
rank lists, 153–54
recruiters, 210–11
relationships
   medical school and,
      64–72, 189
   residency and, 186–90
research
   fellowships, 199
   MD-PhD programs, 16–17,
      52–53, 118–19, 120
   summer, 91, 93–94

residency
  applying to, 146–54
  attendings and, 182–84
  categorical vs. advanced,
      164–66, 167
  changing specialties and,
      177–81
  competition for, 39, 45
  dismissals, 184–85
  drug/alcohol abuse and, 196
  free time and, 191,
      195–96, 197
  goal of, 184
  importance of, 38
  income and, 167
  in-service exams, 181–82
  interviews, 146, 151–52
  osteopathic, 41–42
  pimping, 182
  preparing for, 159–60
  relationships and, 186–90
  sleep deprivation and, 191–92
  special projects and, 184
  starting, 176–77, 186–87
  stress management and, 196
  student loans and, 50–51
  surgical, 178–79
  terminology of, 162–67
  work hour restrictions for,
      192–95
  See also intern year; matching
resume. *See* CV
rolling admissions, 31, 35
rotations
  behavior on, 112–13
  exams and, 115
  goals of, 111–12
  length of, 115
  medicine, 122–30
  pimping and, 115–16
  purpose of, 113–15
  scheduling, 111

sub-internship, 117
surgical, 131–37
rounding, 122–25, 131–32

S
San Francisco Match, 149
scholarships
  MD-PhD, 52–53
  military, 53–55
  sources of, 49
science, enjoyment of, 8
Scrubs (television series), 18, 64
seizures, 126
"Senior AOA" recipients, 108
shelf exams, 115
sleep deprivation, 191–92
SOAP (Supplemental Offer and
      Acceptance Program),
      154
SOAP (subjective, objective,
      assessment, plan)
  notes, 128
specialists vs. generalists, earning
      potential of, 199–200
specialties
  "backup," 155–56
  board certification, 182,
      233–36
  categories of, 122
  changing, 177–81
  choosing, 16, 73–74, 79, 86,
      107–8, 112, 136–37
  competitive, 42, 76, 86,
      102–4, 139–41
  fellowships and, 199–200,
      203–4
  hospital-based, 77
  medicine, 122
  military scholarships and, 54
  MOC and, 250–53
  "nine-to-five," 76–77
  Step 1 scores and, 102–4, 107